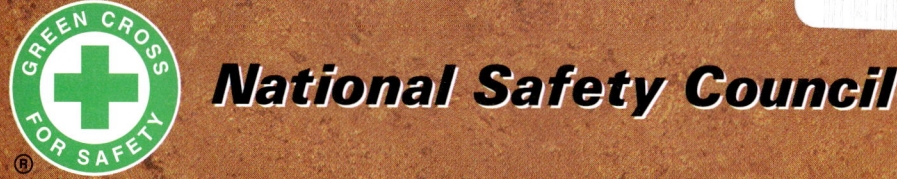

National Safety Council

# INFANT and CHILD CPR

National Safety Council

# INFANT and CHILD CPR

## Jones and Bartlett Publishers
*Sudbury, Massachusetts*

Boston          London          Singapore

*Editorial, Sales, and Customer Service Offices*

Jones and Bartlett Publishers
40 Tall Pine Drive, Sudbury, MA 01776
Internet: http://www.jbpub.com/nsc/, email: nsc@jbpub.com

Jones and Bartlett Publishers International
Barb House, Barb Mews
London W6 7PA, UK

The CPR procedures in this book are based on the most current recommendations of responsible medical sources.  The National Safety Council and the publisher, however, make no guarantee as to, and assume no responsibility for the correctness, sufficiency or completeness of such information or recommendations. Other or additional safety measures may be required under particular circumstances.

**Library of Congress Cataloging-in-Publication Data**
Infant and Child CPR / National Safety Council.
      p.   cm.
   Includes index.
   ISBN 0-7637-0211-0
    1. CPR (First aid) for children.   2. CPR (First aid) for infants.
  I. National Safety Council.
  RJ370.I532   1996
  618.92'1025—dc20                 96-34304
                                   CIP

*Chief Executive Officer:* Clayton E. Jones
*Emergency Care Editor:* Tracy Murphy
*Medical Writer and Author:* Alton L. Thygerson
*Production Administrator:* Anne S. Noonan
*Manufacturing:* Jenna Sturgis
*Editorial Production Service:* Books By Design, Inc.
*Illustrations:* Rolin Graphics
*Typesetting & Pre-press:* Pre-Press Company, Inc.
*Cover Design:* Marshall Henrichs
*Cover Photographs:* Steve Ferry, P & F Communications; Richard Nye
*Printing and Binding:* Banta Company
*Cover Printing:*  Banta Company

Printed in the United States of America
00 99 98 97    10 9 8 7 6 5 4 3 2 1             — 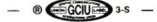 —

# CONTENTS

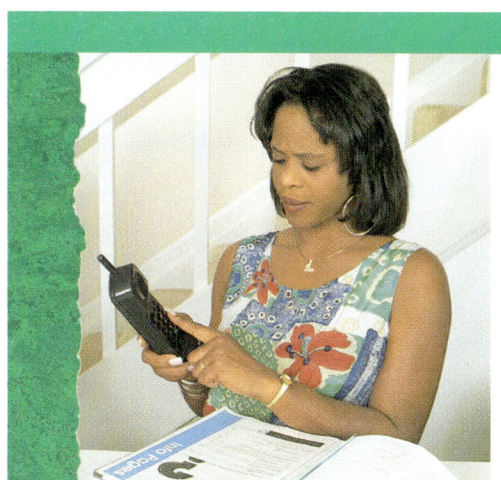

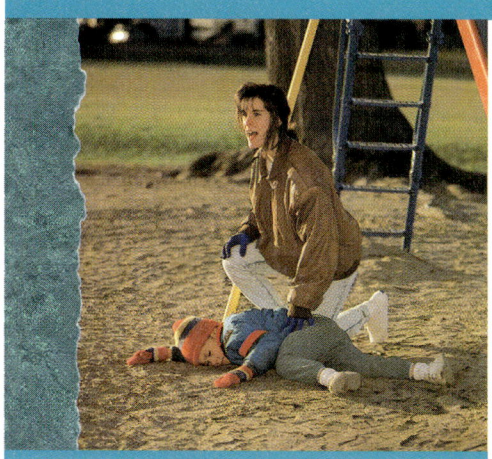

# CONTENTS

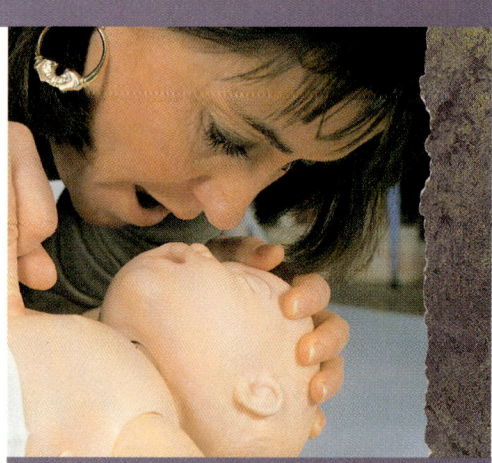

# ABOUT THE NATIONAL SAFETY COUNCIL PROGRAM

**C**ongratulations on selecting the National Safety Council's CPR program! You join good company, as the National Safety Council has successfully trained over 2 million people worldwide in first aid and cardiopulmonary resuscitation (CPR). The National Safety Council's training network of nearly 10,000 instructors at over 2,500 sites worldwide has established the National Safety Council programs as the standard by which all others are judged.

In setting the standards, the National Safety Council has worked in close cooperation with hundreds of national and international organizations, thousands of corporations, thousands of leading educators, dozens of leading medical organizations, and hundreds of state and local governmental agencies. Their collective input has helped create programs that stand alone in quality. Consider just a few of the National Safety Council's current collaborations:

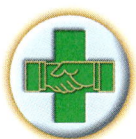

### World's Leading Medical Organizations

The National Safety Council is currently working with both the American Academy of Orthopaedic Surgeons (AAOS) and the Wilderness Medical Society (WMS) to help bring innovative, new training programs to the marketplace. The National Safety Council and the AAOS are developing a new First Responder program and the National Safety Council and the WMS are developing the first-of-its-kind wilderness first aid program.

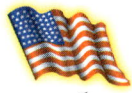

### United States Government

The National Safety Council has developed an innovative computer-based training program for first aid that is currently being used to train United States Postal Service employees.

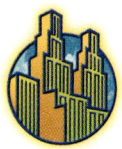

### World's Leading Corporations

Thousands of corporations including Westinghouse, Disney, Exxon, General Motors, Pacific Bell, Ameritech, and U.S. West have selected many of the National Safety Council emergency care programs to train employees.

### World's Leading Colleges and Universities

Hundreds of leading colleges and universities are working closely with the National Safety Council to fully develop and implement the Internet Initiative that will establish the National Safety Council as the leading on-line provider of emergency care programs.

Most importantly, in selecting the National Safety Council programs, you can feel confident that the programs are accepted and approved worldwide. You can rely on the National Safety Council. Founded in 1913, the National Safety Council is dedicated to protecting life, promoting health, and reducing accidental death. For more than 80 years, the National Safety Council has been the world's leading authority on safety/injury education.

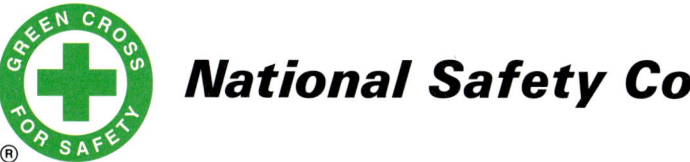

*National Safety Council*

# PART

# 1

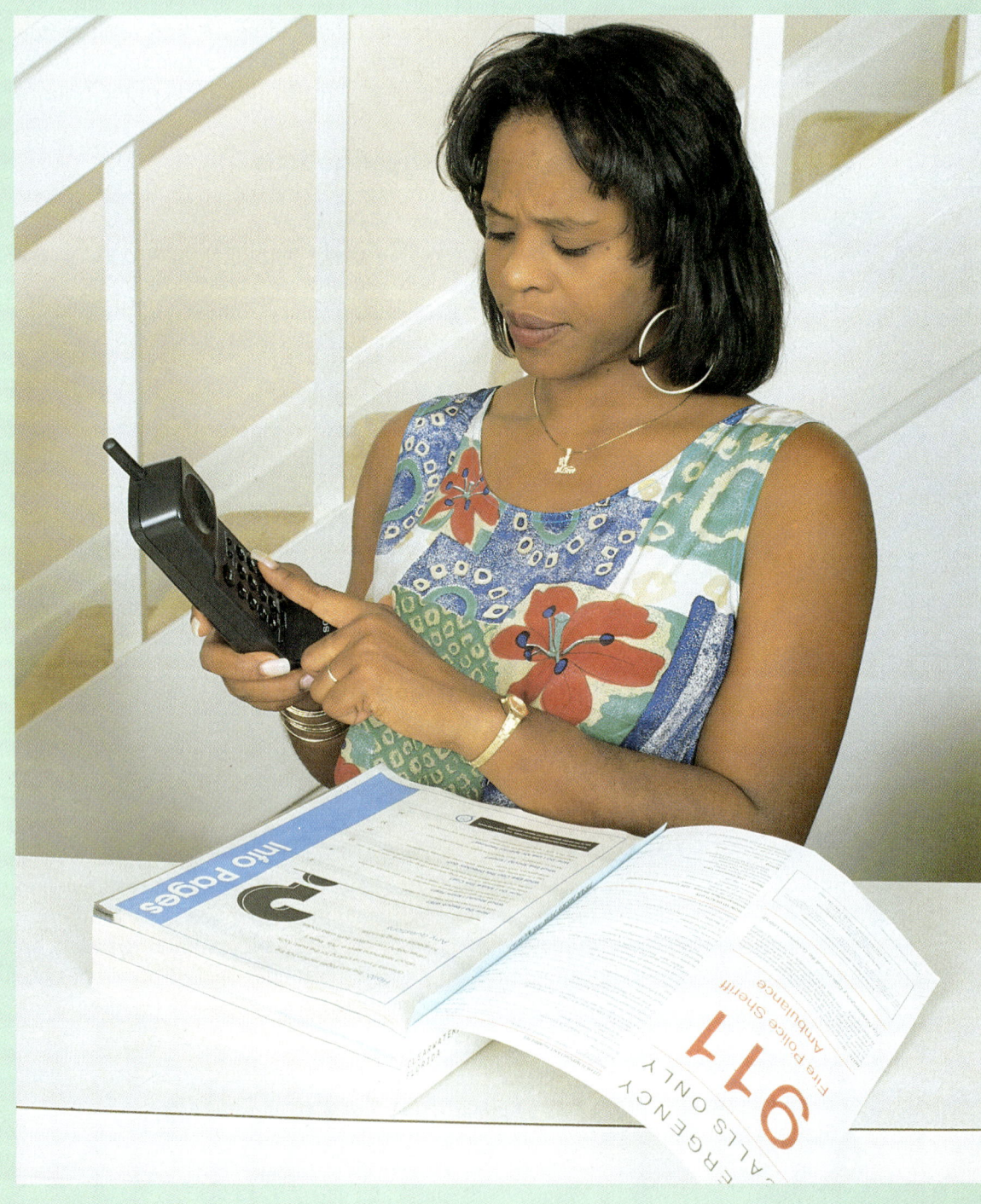

# ACTION AT AN EMERGENCY

## Bystander Intervention

Bystanders are a vital link between the emergency medical service (EMS) and the victim. In order to give a victim the best chance for survival, a bystander must quickly and reliably recognize the emergency and decide to help.

Everyone will at some time have to make a decision whether to help another person. A quick decision to get involved at the time of an emergency is unlikely to occur unless the bystander has considered the possibility of helping in advance. The most important time to make the decision to help is before you encounter an emergency.

Deciding to help is an attitude about helping people in emergencies and about one's competence to deal with emergencies.

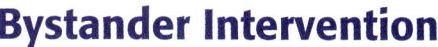

" *Whatever can happen to one man can happen to every man.* "

Lucius Annaeus Seneca (4 B.C.?–A.D. 65)

## Legal Considerations

Legal and ethical issues concern all bystanders. Is a bystander required to stop and give care at an automobile crash? Can a child be treated even when the parents cannot be contacted for their consent? These and many other legal and ethical questions confront bystanders.

### Consent

Before helping, a bystander must gain consent from a victim. Touching another person without his or her permission or consent is unlawful (known as battery) and could be grounds for a lawsuit. Likewise, giving help without the victim's consent is unlawful.

### Expressed Consent

Consent must be obtained from every responsive, mentally competent (i.e., able to make a rational decision) adult (i.e., a person of legal age). If a parent or guardian is nearby, get their permission.

## Implied Consent

Implied consent involves an unresponsive victim and a life-threatening condition. It is assumed or implied that an unresponsive victim would consent to lifesaving interventions. Consent also is implied when the bystander begins care and the victim does not resist.

## Children

Consent must be obtained from a parent or guardian of a child victim, as legally defined by the state. When life-threatening situations exist and the parent or legal guardian is not available for consent, help should be given based on implied consent. Do not withhold help from a minor just to obtain parental or guardian permission.

## Abandonment

**Abandonment** means terminating the care of a victim without ensuring continued care at the same level or higher. Once you have responded to an emergency, you must not leave a victim who needs continuing help until another competent and trained person takes responsibility for the victim. This may seem obvious, but there have been cases in which critically ill or injured victims were left unattended and then died. Thus, a rescuer must stay with the victim until another equally or better trained person takes over.

## Negligence

**Negligence** means deviating from accepted standards of care that results in further injury to the victim. Factors involved in negligence include

1. duty to act
2. breach of duty (substandard care)
3. injury and damages inflicted

## Duty to Act

No one is required to help when no legal duty exists. For example, a physician could ignore a stranger choking or not breathing. While moral obligations may exist, they are not always the same as a legal obligation to help. Duty to act may occur in the following situations:

- *When employment requires it.* If your employer designates you as responsible for rendering first aid to meet Occupational Safety and Health Administration (OSHA) requirements and you are called to an emergency, you have a duty to act. Examples include law enforcement officers, park rangers, athletic trainers, lifeguards, and teachers, all of whose job descriptions designate them to give first aid.
- *When a preexisting responsibility exists.* You may have a preexisting relationship with other persons that demands you be responsible for them, which means you must help if needed. Examples include a parent for a child, a driver for a passenger.

Duty to act means following guidelines for standards of care. Standards of care ensure quality care and protection for injured or suddenly ill victims. The elements that make up standards of care include the following:

- *The type of rescuer.* A rescuer should provide the level and type of care expected of a reasonable person with the same amount of training and in similar circumstances. Different standards of care apply to physicians, nurses, emergency medical technicians (EMTs), and first aiders.
- *Published recommendations.* Emergency care–related organizations and societies publish recommended first aid procedures. For example, the American Heart Association publishes guidelines for giving cardiopulmonary resuscitation (CPR).

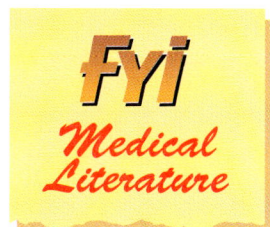

**Chain of Survival** The National Safety Council advocates the Chain of Survival model of emergency cardiac care. The Chain of Survival includes four links: (1) early access; (2) early cardiopulmonary resuscitation (CPR); (3) early defibrillation; and (4) early advanced care. Bystanders are a vital part of the first two links—activation of the EMS and CPR. Skilled EMS personnel provide the other two links—defibrillation and advanced care. A weak or missing link decreases the chance of survival.

1. **Early access.** Early access of the emergency medical service (EMS) enables defibrillation-trained and equipped personnel to arrive at the victim's side more rapidly and enables trained emergency dispatchers to coach bystanders in the provision of CPR until help arrives. The bystander must recognize the emergency, be willing to help, and be able to notify the local EMS.

2. **Early CPR.** Early CPR, which provides rescue breathing and chest compressions, serves as a holding action providing blood and oxygen to vital organs for a few extra minutes until defibrillation and advanced care can be provided. It takes more than CPR to save a life when the heart stops.

   CPR, as we do it today, was first described in 1960. Since then, the technique has changed very little. The earlier it is used, the better. Bystander CPR improves a victim's likelihood of survival. CPR alone has a minimal effect if early defibrillation cannot be provided. Experts claim that poorly performed CPR may be no more effective than no CPR at all.

3. **Early defibrillation.** In most cases of adult cardiac arrest, the heart is in an abnormal rhythm called ventricular fibrillation that can only be reversed by delivering an electrical shock with a machine known as a defibrillator. Each minute delayed for attempted defibrillation reduces the likelihood of survival.

4. **Early advanced care.** Early advanced care includes the three above links plus special care (e.g., intravenous medications) to help stabilize the victim and prevent recurrence of cardiac arrest.

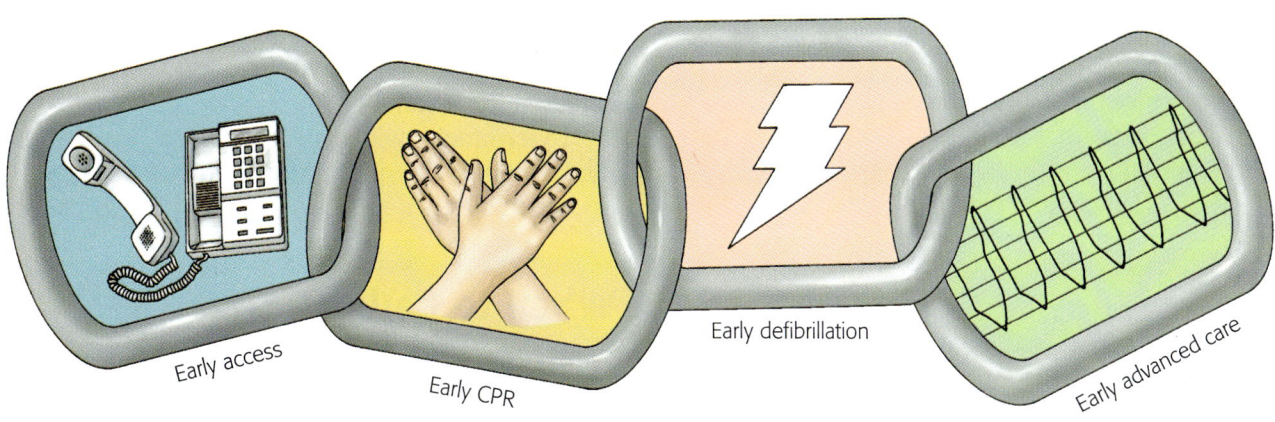

Early access

Early CPR

Early defibrillation

Early advanced care

---

## Breach of Duty

Generally, a rescuer breaches (i.e., "breaks") his or her duty to a victim by failing to provide the type of care as would a person having the same or similar training. There are two ways to breach one's duty: acts of omission and acts of commission. An *act of omission* is the failure to do what a reasonably prudent person with the same or similar training would do in the same or similar circumstances. An *act of commission* is doing something that a reasonably prudent person would *not* do under the same or similar circumstances.

## Injury and Damages Inflicted

Other than physical damage, injury and damage can include physical pain and suffering, mental anguish, medical expenses, and sometimes loss of earnings and earning capacity.

## Confidentiality

Rescuers may become privy to information that would be embarrassing to the victim or the victim's family if it were publicly revealed. It is important that you be extremely cautious about revealing information you learn while caring for someone. The law recognizes that people have the right to privacy.

Do not discuss what you know with anyone other than those who have a medical need to know medical information. State laws require reporting certain incidents such as rape, abuse, and gunshot wounds.

## Good Samaritan Laws

Starting in the early 1960s, a number of states (California was the first, in 1959) enacted laws designed to protect physicians and other medical personnel from legal actions that may arise from emergency treatment they give while not in the line of duty. These laws, known as Good Samaritan laws, encourage people to assist others in distress by granting them immunity against lawsuits. While the laws vary from state to state, Good Samaritan immunity generally applies only when the rescuer is (1) acting during an emergency, (2) acting in good faith, which means he or she has good intentions, (3) acting without compensation, and (4) not guilty of any malicious misconduct or gross negligence toward the victim (deviating from all rational first aid guidelines).

Many legal experts believe that the main effect of Good Samaritan legislation has been to create a false sense of security in the minds of rescuers who erroneously believe that the law protects them from lawsuits regardless of their actions. Good Samaritan laws are easy to get around and should not be looked on as a substitute for competent emergency care and keeping within the scope of your training.

While Good Samaritan laws primarily cover medical personnel, several states have expanded them to include laypersons serving as rescuers. In fact, some states have several Good Samaritan laws that cover different types of people in various situations (e.g., California has 15, New York 8, and Florida 4 different Good Samaritan laws).

Fear of lawsuits has made some people wary of getting involved in emergency situations. Rescuers, however, are rarely sued; for those who are, the courts usually rule in their favor.

## Scene Survey

If you are at the scene of an emergency situation, do a 10-second survey that includes looking for three things: (1) hazards that could be dangerous to you, the victim(s), or bystanders; (2) the mechanism or cause of the injury or injuries; and (3) the number of victims.

As you approach an emergency scene, scan the area for immediate dangers to yourself or to the victim. For example, if an automobile accident has left the involved vehicle in the roadway obstructing traffic, you have to consider whether you can safely go to that vehicle to help the victim. Or you might notice that gasoline is dripping from the gas tank and that the battery has shorted out and is sparking—the car could explode at any moment. In such circumstances you should withdraw and get help before proceeding. You are not being cowardly, merely realistic. Never attempt a rescue that you have not been specifically trained to do. You cannot help another if you also become a victim. Always ask yourself: Is the scene safe to enter?

The second thing to do in the first 10 seconds is to determine the cause of the injury. For example, if the emergency department physician knows that a victim was thrown against a steering wheel, he or she will check for liver, spleen, and cardiac injuries. Be sure to tell the EMS personnel about that, so the physician may initially be able to fully recognize the extent of the injuries.

Determine how many people are injured. There may be more than one victim, so look around and ask about others involved.

## When to Call the EMS

Generally you will know when an emergency happens. You can tell by the type of injuries or by how the victim looks that it is time to call for help. Call the EMS whenever a situation is more than you can handle. In the following instances, calling the EMS is definitely the right thing to do:

- severe bleeding
- drowning
- electrocution
- breathing difficulty or no breathing
- choking
- altered mental status
- poisoning

**Do a 10-second scene survey by looking for three things:**

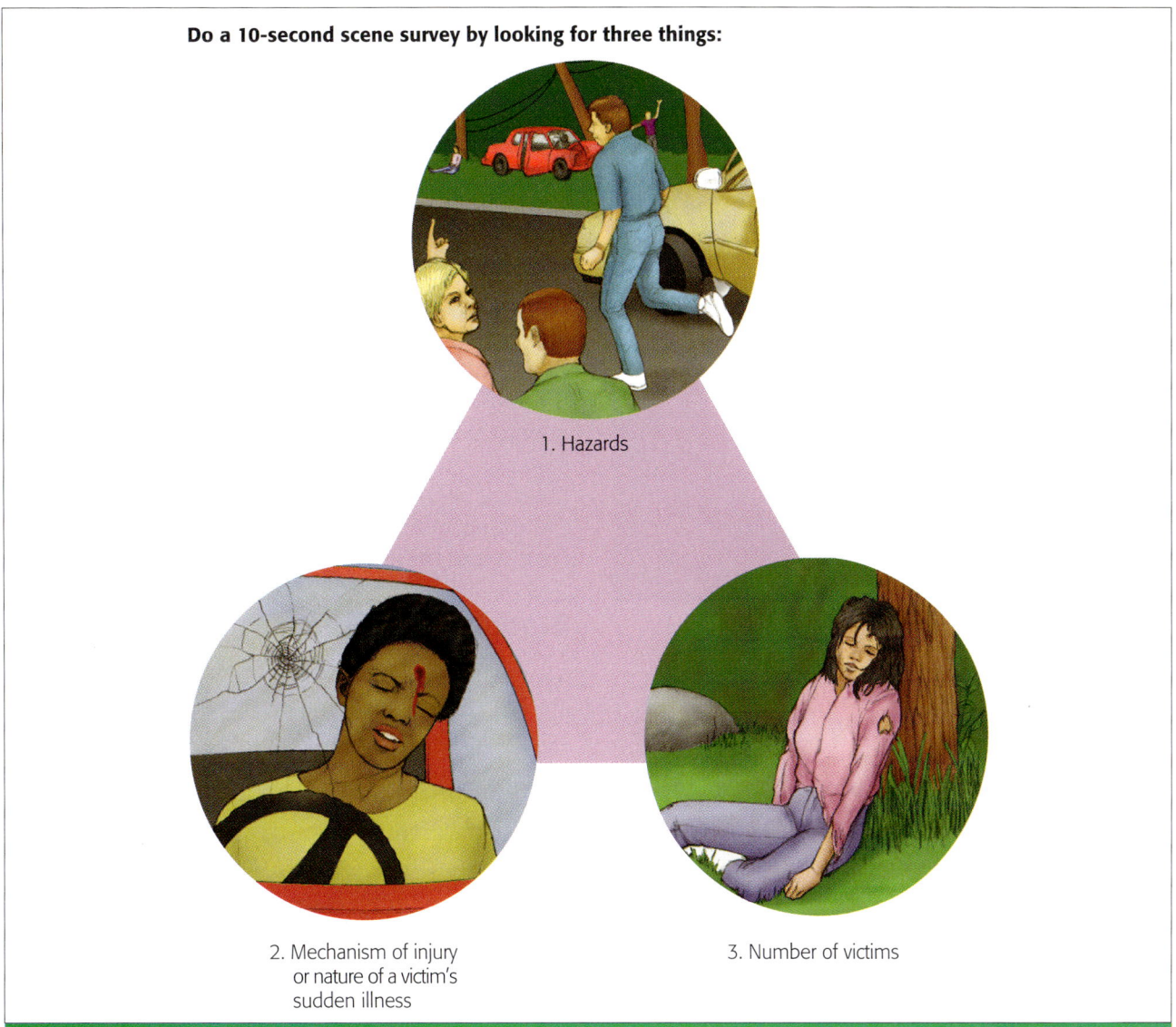

1. Hazards

2. Mechanism of injury or nature of a victim's sudden illness

3. Number of victims

Scene Survey

- some seizure cases (most do not require EMS assistance)
- no pulse
- critical burns
- spine injury

## How to Call the EMS

To receive emergency assistance of every kind in most communities, you simply phone 911. Check to see if this is true in your community. Emergency telephone numbers usually are listed on the inside front cover of all telephone directories. Keep these numbers near or on every telephone. Call "O" (the operator) if you do not know the emergency number.

If you have to call the EMS, be ready to give the dispatcher the following information. Speak slowly and clearly.

1. The victim's location. Give the address, names of intersecting roads, and other landmarks, if possible. This information is the most important you can give. Also, tell the specific location of the victim (e.g., "in the basement").
2. Your phone number and name. This prevents false calls and allows a dispatch center without the enhanced 911 system to call back for additional information, if needed.
3. What happened. State the nature of the emergency (e.g., "My child won't wake up").

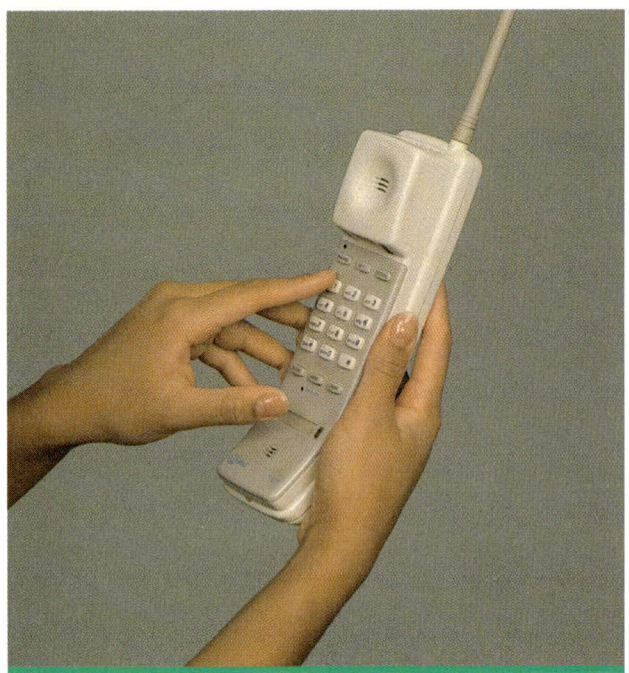

For help, phone 911 or the local emergency number.

4. Number of persons needing help and any special conditions.
5. Victim's condition (e.g., "My child is not breathing") and any emergency care you have tried (such as rescue breathing).

Do *not* hang up the phone unless the dispatcher instructs you to do so. Enhanced 911 systems can track a call, but some communities lack this technology or are still using a seven-digit emergency number. Also, the EMS dispatcher may tell you how to best care for the victim. If you send someone else to call, have the person report back to you so you can be sure the call was made. Other tips include:

- Teach children what 911 is for and how and when to call. Refer to "nine-one-one," not "nine-eleven," because children may expect to find an 11 on the dial or on the push buttons.
- Do not hang up without explanation if 911 is called by mistake, or the dispatcher will have to call back to see if you need help.
- If your area does not have a 911 system, add EMS, fire, and police numbers to a list by your phones. During an emergency, you may not have the time or presence of mind to find a number in a directory.

When a serious situation occurs, call the EMS (911 in most communities) *first.* Do *not* call your doctor, the hospital, a friend, relatives, or neighbors for help before you call the EMS. Calling anyone else first only wastes time.

If the situation is not an emergency, call your doctor. However, if you are in *any* doubt as to whether the situation is an emergency, call the EMS.

## Disease Precautions

Rescuers must be aware of the risks associated with emergency medical care. One such risk comes from infectious diseases, which can range in severity from mild to life threatening. Rescuers should know how to reduce the risk of contamination to themselves and to others. This section stresses the importance of precautionary measures that help to protect against infection from disease agents such as viruses and bacteria.

### Bloodborne Disease

Some diseases are caused by microorganisms that are "borne" (carried) in a person's bloodstream. Contact with blood infected with such microorganisms may cause infection. Of the many bloodborne pathogens, three pose significant health threats to rescuers: hepatitis B virus (HBV), hepatitis C virus, and human immunodeficiency virus (HIV).

#### Hepatitis B

Each year, as many as 12,000 people come down with hepatitis B, the most common form of hepatitis. Hepatitis is a viral infection of the liver. Types A, B, and C are seen most often. Each is caused by a different virus.

A vaccine for hepatitis B is available and is recommended for all infants and for adults who may have contact with carriers of the disease or with blood. Medical and laboratory workers, police, intravenous drug users, people with multiple sexual partners, and those living with someone who has lifelong infection are at high risk of hepatitis B (and hepatitis C as well). Vaccination is the best defense against HBV. There is no chance of developing hepatitis B from the vaccine. Federal laws require employers to offer a series of three vaccine injections free to all employees who may be at risk of exposure.

Without vaccination shots, exposure to hepatitis B may produce symptoms within two weeks to six months following exposure. People with hepatitis B infection may be symptom free, but that does *not* mean they are not contagious. These people may infect others through exposure to their blood. Symptoms of hepatitis B resemble those of the flu and include fatigue, nausea, loss of appetite, stomach pain, and perhaps a yellowing of the skin.

Hepatitis B starts as an inflammation of the liver and usually lasts one to two months. In a few people, the infection is very serious, and in some, mild infection continues for life. The virus may stay in the liver and can lead to severe damage (cirrhosis) and liver cancer. Medical treatment that begins immediately after exposure may prevent infection from developing.

## Hepatitis C

Hepatitis C, first identified in the 1980s, is caused by a different virus from HBV, but both diseases have a great deal in common. Like hepatitis B, hepatitis C affects the liver and can lead to long-term liver disease and liver cancer. Hepatitis C varies in severity and may even cause no symptoms at the time of infection. Currently, there is no vaccine or effective treatment for hepatitis C.

## HIV

Estimates are that over 1.5 million people in the United States are infected with HIV but have no symptoms. A person infected with HIV can infect others, and HIV-infected persons almost always develop acquired immunodeficiency syndrome (AIDS), which interferes with the body's ability to fight off other diseases. No vaccine is available to prevent HIV infection, which eventually proves fatal. Since 1981, more than 250,000 Americans have died of AIDS-related illnesses. It is predicted that by the year 2000, the majority of those afflicted with HIV will be females and children. The best defense against AIDS is to avoid becoming infected.

## How Bloodborne Pathogens Are Transmitted

HIV and HBV are usually transmitted (passed on) when disease organisms in body fluids enter the body through mucous membranes or through breaks in the skin. The most common forms of transmission are:

- sexual contact with an infected person
- from an infected mother to her unborn child
- sharing needles with infected intravenous drug users

A rescuer may be exposed through an open sore or wound that comes in contact with a victim's infectious blood or other body fluids that contain blood or when the rescuer is not wearing the proper personal protective equipment (PPE) to protect against contact with infectious material.

## Protection

In most cases, you can control the risk of exposure to bloodborne pathogens by wearing the proper PPE and by following some simple procedures.

### Personal Protective Equipment (PPE)

This equipment blocks entry of an organism into the body. The most common type of protection is gloves. The Food and Drug Administration (FDA), the Centers for Disease Control and Prevention (CDC), and the Occupational Safety and Health Administration (OSHA) have stated that vinyl and latex gloves are equally protective. Research indicates that latex has fewer micropores (very small holes) and thus offers the most protection. However, latex tends to break down faster over time (several years) while they may be in a first aid kit, waiting to be used. All first aid kits should have several pairs of gloves.

Protective eyewear and a standard surgical mask may be necessary at some emergencies; rescuers ordinarily will not have or need such equipment.

Mouth-to-barrier devices are recommended for rescue breathing and CPR. No case of disease transmission to a rescuer as a result of performing unprotected CPR on an infected victim has been documented. Nevertheless, a mouth-to-barrier device should be used whenever possible.

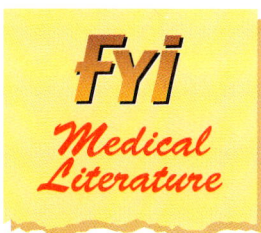

**Do Gloves Really Protect?** A study tested the effectiveness of vinyl and latex gloves as barriers to hand contamination. Gloves were checked according to the American Society for Testing and Materials and leaks occurred with 43 percent of vinyl gloves and 9 percent of latex gloves. The researchers concluded that latex gloves, and to a lesser extent vinyl gloves, provide substantial protection during hand contact with moist body substances, functioning as a barrier even when leaks are present. Since leaks are not always detected by the wearer, hand washing should routinely follow the use of disposable gloves.

*Source:* R. J. Olsen et al., "Examination Gloves as Barriers to Hand Contamination in Clinical Practice." *Journal of the American Medical Association,* 270:350–53 (1993).

## Universal Precautions or Body Substance Isolation?

Individuals infected with HBV or HIV may not show symptoms and may not even know they are infectious. For that reason, all human blood and body fluids should be considered infectious, and precautions should be taken to avoid contact. The *body substance isolation* (BSI) technique assumes that *all* body fluids are a possible risk. EMS personnel routinely follow BSI procedures, even if blood or body fluids are not visible.

OSHA requires any company with employees who are expected to give help in an emergency to follow *universal precautions,* which assume that *all* blood and *certain* body fluids pose a risk for transmission of HBV and HIV. OSHA considers an employee who assists another with a nosebleed or a cut to fall under the definition of "Good Samaritan." Such acts, however, are not considered occupational exposure unless the employee who provides the assistance is a member of a first aid team or is designated or expected to render first aid as part of his or her job. In essence, OSHA's requirement excludes unassigned employees who perform unanticipated first aid.

Whenever there is a chance you could be exposed to bloodborne pathogens, your employer must provide appropriate PPE, which might include eye protection, gloves, gowns, and masks. The PPE must be accessible, and your employer must provide training to help you choose the right PPE for your work.

While EMS personnel follow BSI procedures and OSHA requires designated worksite rescuers to follow universal precautions, what should a typical rescuer do? It makes sense for rescuers to follow BSI procedures and assume that *all* blood and body fluids are infectious and follow appropriate protective measures.

## Coping with Emergencies

When an injury occurs, rescuers can protect themselves and others against bloodborne pathogens by following these steps:

1. Wear appropriate PPE, such as gloves and mouth-to-barrier devices.
2. If you have been trained in the correct procedures, use absorbent barriers to soak up blood or other infectious materials.
3. Clean the spill area with an appropriate disinfecting solution, such as diluted bleach.

4. Discard contaminated materials in an appropriate waste disposal container.

If you have been exposed to blood or body fluids:

1. Use soap and water to wash the parts of your body that have been contaminated.
2. If the exposure happens while at work, report the incident to your supervisor. Otherwise, contact your personal physician. Early action can prevent the development of hepatitis B and enable affected workers to track potential HIV infection.

The best protection against bloodborne disease is using the safeguards described here. By following these guidelines, rescuers can decrease their chance of contracting bloodborne illness.

## Airborne Disease

Infective organisms (e.g., bacteria, viruses) that are introduced into the air by coughing or sneezing are said to be "airborne." Droplets of mucus that carry those bacteria or viruses can then be inhaled by other individuals. The rate of tuberculosis (TB) has increased recently and is receiving much attention. TB, caused by bacteria, sometimes settles in the lungs and can be fatal. In most cases, a rescuer will not know that a victim has TB. Assume that any person with a cough, especially one who is in a nursing home or a shelter, may have TB. Other symptoms include fatigue, weight loss, chest pain, and coughing up blood. If a surgical mask is available, wear it or wrap a handkerchief over your nose and mouth.

### Glove Removal

Proper glove removal is as important as wearing gloves to protect against infection. Follow this procedure:

1. Grip one glove near the cuff and peel it down until it comes off inside out. Cup it in the palm of your gloved hand.
2. Place two fingers of your bare hand inside the cuff of the remaining glove.
3. Peel that glove down so it also comes off inside out and over the first glove.
4. Properly dispose of the gloves.
5. Wash your hands with soap and water.

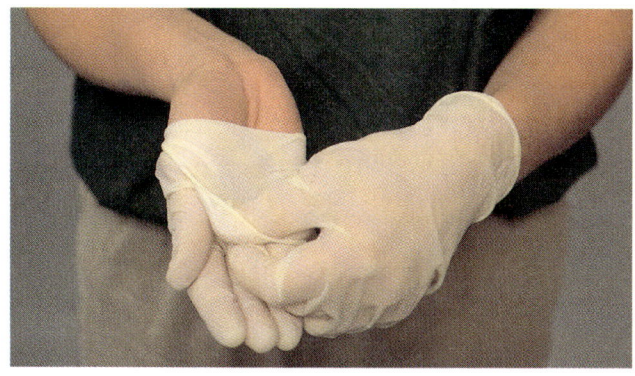

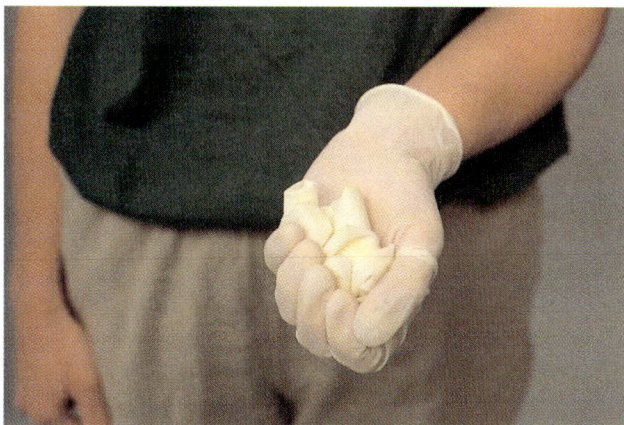

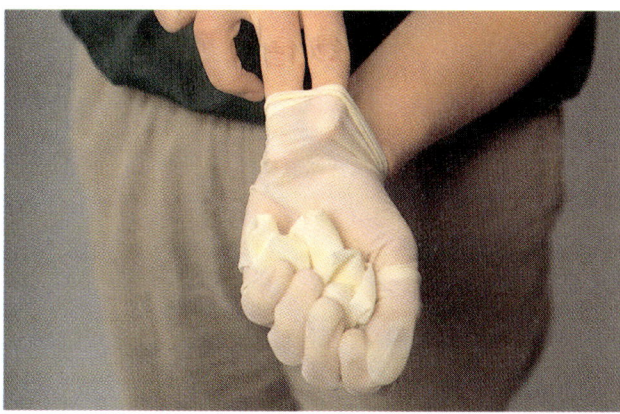

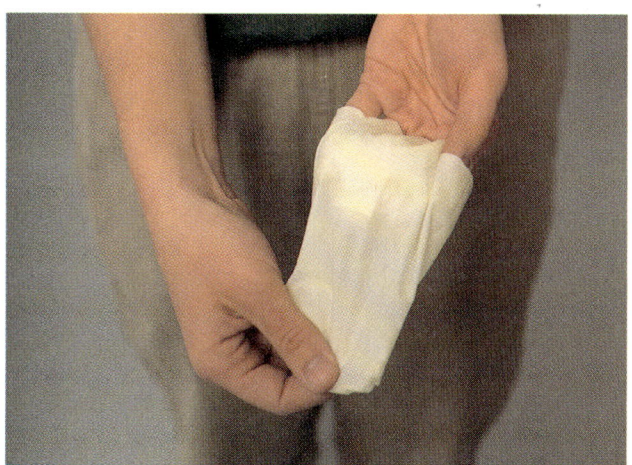

Glove removal

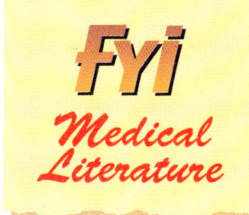

## CPR Training and HIV

With concerns about the human immunodeficiency virus (HIV) and other infectious agents, many people are wondering whether disinfection procedures are adequate to prevent the transmission of diseases by way of manikins used for CPR training. A report suggests that even less-than-thorough disinfection with 70-percent isopropyl alcohol is enough to prevent the spread of the virus that causes AIDS. In fact, the study suggests that just wiping the manikin with a dry cloth may be sufficient.

Although there have been no cases to date of HIV transmitted by CPR manikins, the virus is found in saliva and can survive for a time on plastic material. And other diseases, such as herpes, have been contracted during CPR training. While the risk is minimal, it is important to ease fears about disease transmission if widespread CPR training nationwide is to be promoted.

The currently preferred method of disinfecting equipment is to use a bleach solution, with isopropyl alcohol available as an option. When isopropyl alcohol is used, it is supposed to be applied to the manikin for 60 seconds. To test the effectiveness of these agents, the researchers applied a concentrated dose of HIV-infected white blood cells—a much denser concentration than would be found in saliva—to the face mask of a CPR manikin. They then used alcohol to disinfect the manikin, but they disinfected for only 5 or 10 seconds. They also looked at the effects of simply wiping with a dry cloth. After each cleaning, the researchers checked the manikin to determine whether any infected white blood cells remained.

The study reported that even with sloppy cleaning, decontamination was effective. "Our data suggest that one should not refrain from CPR training out of fear of contracting HIV infection," the researchers concluded.

*Source:* I. B. Corless, A. Lisker, R. W. Buckheit, "Decontamination of an HIV-contaminated CPR Manikin," American Journal of Public Health 82:1542–1543 (1992).

# Checking the Victim

During emergency situations, when panic is likely to exist, knowing what to do and what *not* to do can be vital. Effective care depends on effective assessment—you need to find what is wrong before you can treat it.

The saying "first things first" may seem obvious in most emergency situations, but it is not always obvious which injuries take precedence. A logical, systematic format known as **victim assessment** will help you evaluate the situation.

After you have determined that the situation is safe (see page 6), you can perform the primary survey. Make all assessments while kneeling close to the victim.

If two or more people are injured, attend to the quiet one first. A quiet victim may not have an open airway or a pulse. A victim who is talking, crying, or yelling obviously has an open airway.

## The Primary Survey

The respiratory and circulatory systems are two of the most important organs in the body. A serious problem in either body system generally produces a serious threat to life. And if either system stops functioning, death occurs within minutes.

The goal of the primary survey is to quickly assess two of the most important body systems. The heart and lungs are essential to life. Any life-threatening condition, such as an obstructed airway, must be corrected before you continue the victim assessment. Since most injured victims won't have life-threatening conditions, most primary surveys will be completed quickly.

The first step in caring for any victim is to find the most life-threatening conditions. Always assess and care for the three most important body systems in the "ABC" order of importance:

- Respiratory system
  **A**: **A**irway open?
  **B**: **B**reathing?
- Circulatory system
  **C**: **C**irculation (Pulse? Hemorrhage? Skin condition?)

Give priority to caring for the ABCs for lifesaving care. When dealing with injured victims, you may need to remove some of a victim's clothing to complete the assessment.

Form a general impression of the victim based on an immediate assessment of the scene. Look at the surroundings and the mechanism of injury for an injured victim. Then assess the victim's responsiveness or mental status. If you suspect a spine injury, stabilize the spine.

## A: Open the Airway

If the victim is talking or responsive, the airway is open. For an unresponsive victim, open the airway with the head-tilt/chin-lift method unless you suspect a spine injury (see pages 18 and 25).

## B: Assess Breathing

Responsive victims are breathing. Note any breathing difficulties or unusual breathing sounds such as wheezing, crowing, gurgling, or snoring. If the victim is unresponsive, keep the airway open and look for the chest to rise and fall, listen for breathing, and feel for air coming out of the victim's nose and mouth. If there is no breathing, give two breaths. If an unresponsive victim is breathing, place the victim on his or her left side (**recovery position**). Refer to page 15 for details.

## C: Assess Circulation

Check an unresponsive victim's pulse by feeling at the side of the neck (carotid artery) or, for an infant, at the upper arm (brachial artery). If a pulse is absent, cardiopulmonary resuscitation (CPR) is required. If a pulse is present, but there is no breathing, give rescue breathing. Refer to pages 19 and 26 for details.

## Clothing

Clothing can hide an injury. How much clothing you should remove varies, depending on the victim's condition and injuries. The general rule is to remove as much clothing as necessary to determine the presence or absence of a condition or an injury. Keep in mind that most injured victims are susceptible to hypothermia. If the removal of certain items of clothing may prove embarrassing to the victim or to bystanders, explain what you intend to do and why.

For emergencies involving basic life support, remove or loosen clothing if:

- collar does not allow feeling the carotid pulse
- heavy clothing hinders locating the notch at the sternum's tip, or
- you are unable to find the correct hand position

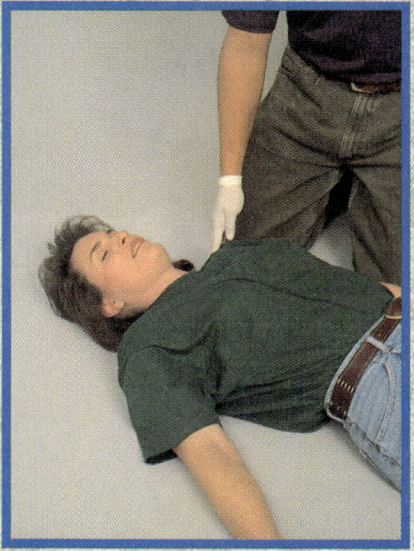

1.

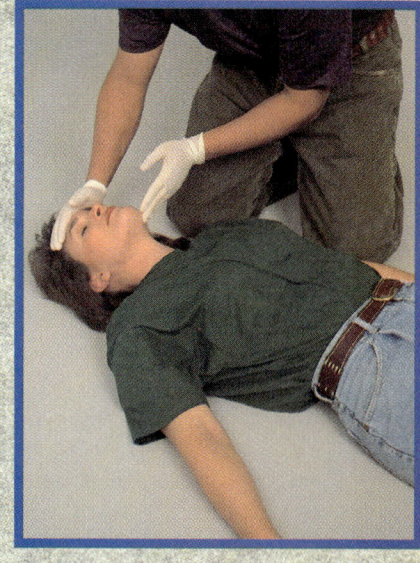

2.

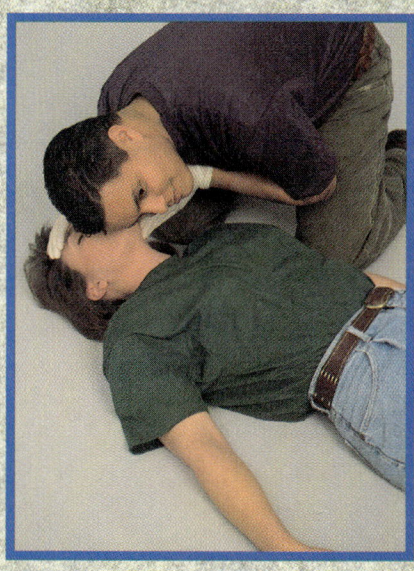

3.

4

**1.** Responsive? Victim's mental status—use AVPU scale

**2.** A = Airway open?

**3.** B = Breathing?

**4.** C = Circulation; carotid pulse?

# PRIMARY SURVEY

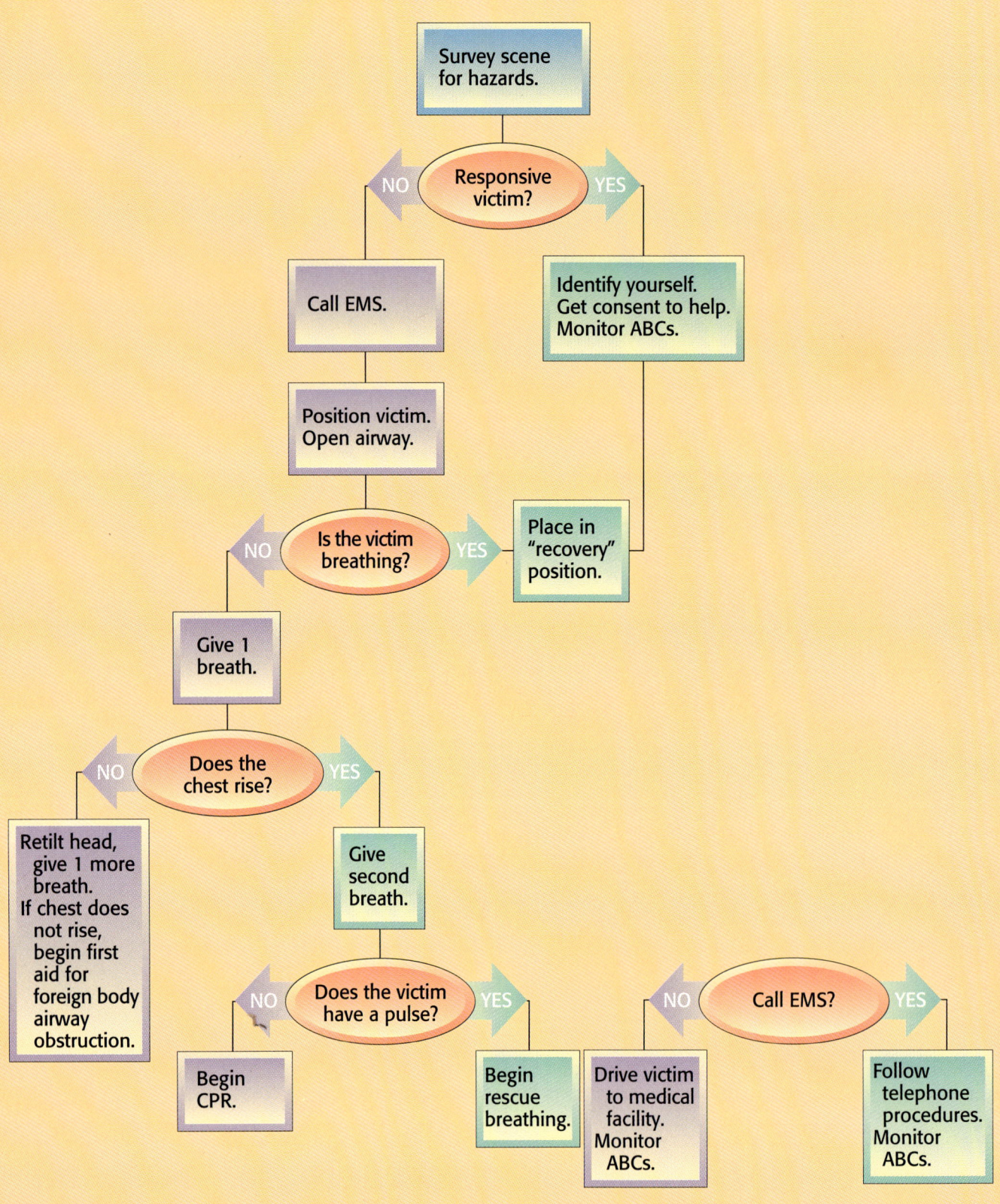

Survey scene for hazards.

Responsive victim?

**NO** → Call EMS. → Position victim. Open airway.

**YES** → Identify yourself. Get consent to help. Monitor ABCs.

Is the victim breathing?

**NO** → Give 1 breath.

**YES** → Place in "recovery" position.

Does the chest rise?

**NO** → Retilt head, give 1 more breath. If chest does not rise, begin first aid for foreign body airway obstruction.

**YES** → Give second breath.

Does the victim have a pulse?

**NO** → Begin CPR.

**YES** → Begin rescue breathing.

Drive victim to medical facility. Monitor ABCs.

Call EMS?

**NO** → Drive victim to medical facility. Monitor ABCs.

**YES** → Follow telephone procedures. Monitor ABCs.

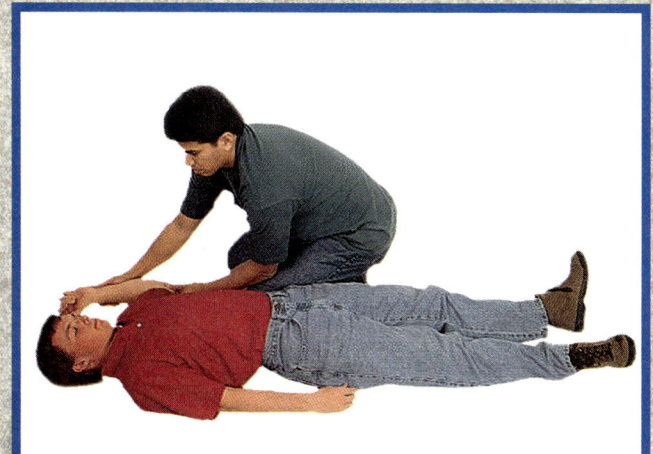

1.

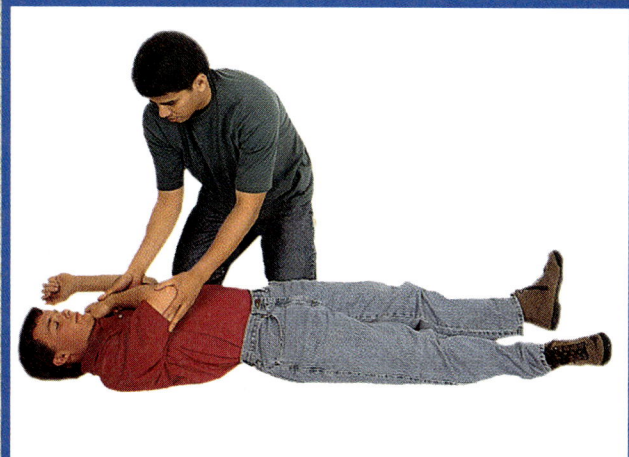

2.

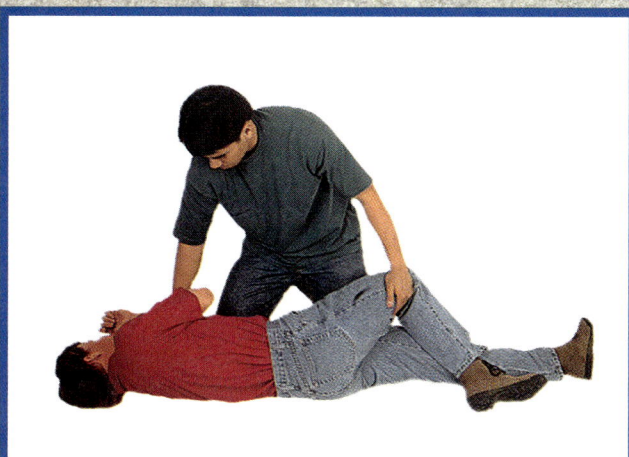

3.

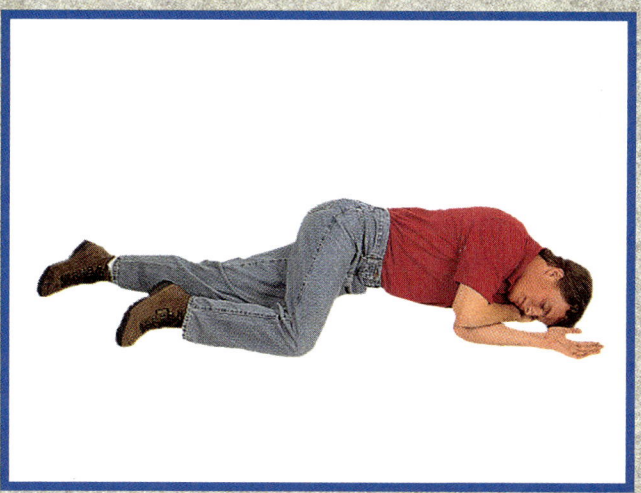

4.

**1.** Bend arm. Keep legs straight.

**2.** Place back of victim's hand against cheek and hold there.

**3.** Hold victim's hand against cheek to support head. Pull bent legs and roll victim toward you.

**4.** Hand supports head. Bent knee prevents rolling. Bent arm gives stability. Front view of recovery position.

# PART

# 2

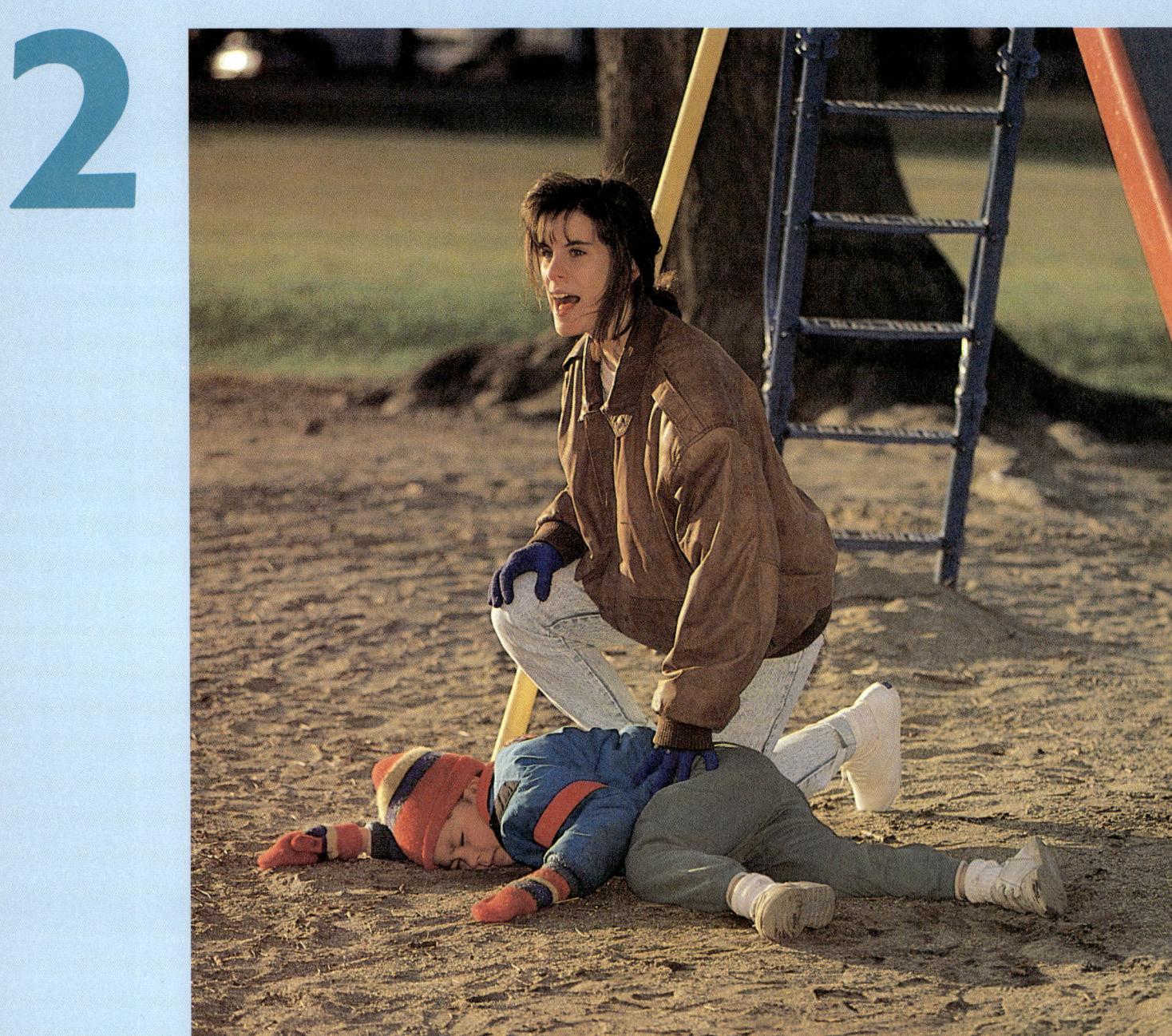

# CHILD BASIC LIFE SUPPORT*

## Child Rescue Breathing and CPR

For the nonbreathing child (one to eight years old), rescue breathing must be started immediately. This is one of the most important procedures that you as a rescuer will be called on to do. For best results, you must understand the process so well that you can proceed automatically.

### Check Responsiveness

The first step is to recognize that a child is unresponsive. The simplest method to determine unresponsiveness is to tap the child's shoulder and shout, "Are you okay?" Do not forcefully shake the child, since he or she may have a spine injury.

### Position the Unconscious Child

An unresponsive child lying facedown must be turned over so CPR can be given, if necessary. If you must turn the child over, keep the head, neck, and shoulders aligned to avoid any twisting of the body. To turn an unresponsive child, follow these steps:

1. Kneel at the child's side.
2. Raise the child's arm closest to you.
3. Adjust the child's legs so they are nearly straight (crossing the ankles helps).
4. Support the head and neck with one hand.
5. Reach over to the child's outside hip and grasp clothing or the edge of the hip with your other hand.
6. Turn the child as a complete unit, pulling steadily and evenly to roll him or her toward you.

### Activate EMS

After determining unresponsiveness, direct another person to activate the EMS (usually by telephoning 911). If you are alone, activate the EMS yourself after

*Based on the American Heart Association, Guidelines for Cardiopulmonary Resuscitation and Emergency Cardiac Care, *JAMA* 268:2172 (1992).

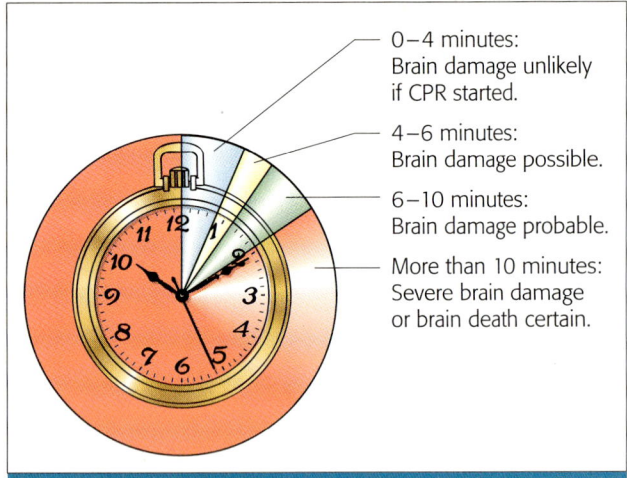

0–4 minutes:
Brain damage unlikely
if CPR started.

4–6 minutes:
Brain damage possible.

6–10 minutes:
Brain damage probable.

More than 10 minutes:
Severe brain damage
or brain death certain.

Start resuscitation efforts at once. Brain damage occcurs without oxygen.

one minute of resuscitation. Do this in the least amount of time possible.

## Open the Airway

The most important maneuver in performing rescue breathing is opening the child's airway. The most common cause of airway obstruction in an unconscious person is blockage by the tongue. When a child's airway is opened, the lower jaw is moved forward, bringing the base of the tongue (which is attached to the lower jaw) forward also and away from the back of the throat. The easiest way to open an injured child's airway is by tilting the head and lifting the chin, however, children's airways have more pliable tissues and are at greater risk for hyperextension of their necks. Perform this maneuver carefully.

To perform the head-tilt/chin-lift, place one hand, palm down, on the victim's forehead and push downward so the head tilts back. Then place the index and middle fingers of your other hand under the lower edge of the chin to lift the jaw. Simply opening the child's airway sometimes results in restoration of breathing.

If you suspect a spine injury, first try to open the airway by lifting the chin without tilting the head back. If the airway remains blocked, tilt the head slowly and gently until the airway is open. Another technique for a child with a possible spine injury is to use a jaw thrust without a head tilt. While stabilizing the head, place the fingers of each hand behind the angles of the child's lower jaw on each side of the head and move the lower jaw forward without tilting the head backward. If the air-

way does not open, it may be necessary to tilt the head slightly.

## Check for Breathing

After determining unresponsiveness and opening the airway, the next step is to look, listen, and feel for breathing. *Look* to see whether there is any visible movement of the child's chest, *listen* for air by placing your ear next to the child's mouth and nose, and *feel* for air by placing your cheek next to the child's mouth and nose. If breathing is present, you will see the child's chest rise and fall, hear air coming from the child's mouth and nose, and feel air against your cheek. This process should take only three to five seconds. Place a breathing unconscious child in the recovery position.

## Perform Rescue Breathing

If a child is not breathing, perform rescue breathing by using one of the following methods: mouth to mouth, mouth to nose, or mouth to barrier device.

### Mouth-to-Mouth Method

The mouth-to-mouth method of rescue breathing is the simplest, quickest, and most effective method for an emergency situation.

During rest, a child's breathing rate is about 20 times per minute (which is enough to sustain life). Exhaled air is about 16 percent oxygen in comparison to room air, which is 21 percent.

Mouth-to-mouth breathing is preferred over mouth-to-nose breathing, especially if there is nasal

### How a Child and Infant Differ from an Adult

- Small airways are easily blocked by secretions and airway swelling.
- Tongue is large relative to small jaw and can block airway in an unresponsive child or infant.
- Infants are nose breathers; removing a secretion can improve breathing problems in an infant.
- Airways have more pliable tissues—be careful not to hyperextend the neck when positioning the airway.
- Risk of hypothermia is greater.

bleeding, injury, or blockage. To perform mouth-to-mouth rescue breathing, follow these steps:

1. Make sure the child's head is positioned with the neck extended and the head tilted backward to open the airway (do not hyperextend the neck).
2. Pinch the child's nose closed to prevent air from escaping, using the same hand that is on the child's forehead to keep the neck extended.
3. Take a breath.
4. Make a tight seal with your mouth around the child's mouth.
5. Slowly blow air into the child's mouth until you see the chest rise.
6. Remove your mouth to allow the air to come out and turn your head away as you take another breath.
7. Repeat one more breath.

If the first breath does not go in, retilt the child's head and try a second breath. If the second breath does not go in, go to the section on unconscious choking management on pages 31 and 33.

### Mouth-to-Nose Method

Although mouth-to-mouth breathing is successful in the majority of cases, certain complications necessitate mouth-to-nose rescue breathing: the child's mouth cannot be opened, a good seal cannot be made around the child's mouth, the child's mouth is severely injured, or the child has no teeth.

The mouth-to-nose technique is performed like mouth-to-mouth breathing, except that you force your exhaled breath through the child's nose while holding his or her mouth closed with one hand pushing up on the chin. The child's mouth then must be held open so any nasal obstruction does not impede exhalation of air from the child's lungs.

### Mouth-to-Barrier Device

A mouth-to-barrier device is an apparatus that is placed over a child's face as a safety precaution for the rescuer during rescue breathing. There are two types of mouth-to-barrier devices:

- *Face masks.* Face masks cover the child's mouth and nose. Most have a one-way valve so exhaled air from the child does not enter the rescuer's mouth. According to the American Heart Association, face masks are more effective than face shields.
- *Face shields.* These clear plastic devices have a mouthpiece through which the rescuer

## Advantages of the Left-Side Position

Left-side positioning is referred to by several terms: recovery position, left lateral recumbent position, left lateral decubitus position, and stable-side position. Positioning a person on his or her left side has several advantages:

- It keeps the airway open in an unresponsive breathing victim without a spine injury.
- It protects the lungs from aspiration should vomiting occur.
- It delays vomiting by placing the esophagus above the stomach.
- It delays a poison's effects by retaining the poison in the stomach (the pyloric sphincter is kept straight up). A poison can be better dealt with in the stomach than in the small intestine.

breathes. Some models have a short airway that is inserted into the child's mouth over the tongue. They are smaller and less expensive than face masks, but air can leak around the shield. Also, they cover only the child's mouth, so the nose must be pinched. The American Heart Association recommends replacing face shields with face masks as soon as possible.

Use of a barrier device requires the child's neck to be tilted and the chin lifted. After the mask is in place, the rescuer breathes through the device. The technique is performed like mouth-to-mouth breathing.

## Check for a Pulse

After you have given the first two breaths, locate the child's pulse to see if the heart is beating. To find the pulse, maintain the head-tilt position with one hand pushing backward on the child's forehead and use the tips of the index and the middle fingers of your other hand to locate the child's Adam's apple (larynx or voice box). Then slide the two fingers into the groove between the Adam's apple and the muscle at the side of the neck for the carotid pulse.

Feel for the carotid artery on the side of the child's neck closer to you. You should not feel for the carotid artery on the far side of the child's neck for two reasons: (1) there is a greater tendency to apply unnecessary pressure on the trachea, which can obstruct the airway, and (2) there is a greater

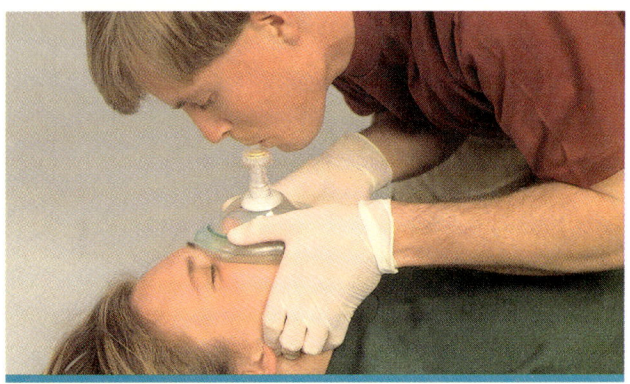

Mouth-to-barrier device

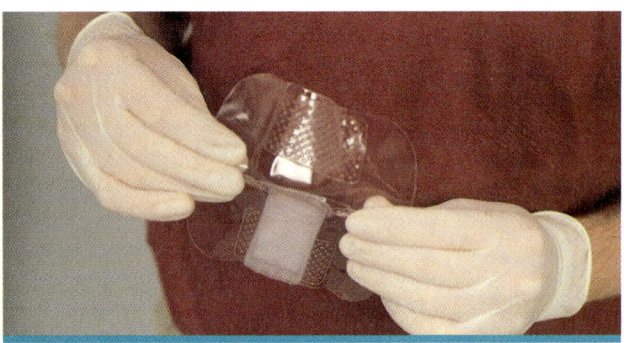

Face shield

tendency to feel for the pulse by using your thumb and feeling both sides of the neck simultaneously. Feeling with the thumb, which has its own pulse, can give a false indication of a pulse in the child.

The reasons for feeling the carotid pulse are that it is immediately accessible and you are already positioned at the child's head and neck. Also, a felt carotid pulse will persist when other pulses (e.g., radial pulse) cannot be detected. Locating the carotid pulse is easily learned.

Feel for the carotid artery gently and without undue pressure. It should take 5 to 10 seconds to feel for the pulse, except in cases of hypothermia, when 30 to 45 seconds should be taken.

If the child has no pulse, CPR must be started immediately.

If the child has a pulse but is not breathing, continue rescue breathing at a rate of one breath every 3 seconds, or 20 times per minute. Between breaths, remove your mouth to take a breath and to permit air to flow out of the child's lungs. As you remove your mouth, turn your head toward the child's feet to see whether the child's chest falls after each breath. A method for timing the breaths for every three seconds is to breathe into the child for

about one second, count "one–one thousand," then take a breath for yourself on the third second. After 20 breaths, recheck the child's pulse and breathing.

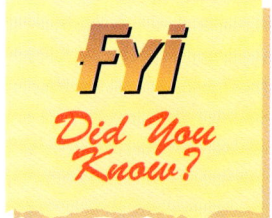

Arteries received their name (from the Greek for *windpipe*) because the Greek physician Praxagoras thought they carried air. (In corpses they are usually empty and that was probably where his observations were made.)

The carotid arteries along the neck convey the blood to the head, and if pressure is applied to them, the individual drops off into a stupor or slumbers. Hence, the Greeks called these arteries the "karotides" from the Greek word *karoun*, meaning "to stupefy."

*Source:* Skinner, Henry A., *The Origin of Medical Terms*, 2nd edition (Baltimore: Williams and Wilkins).

## Perform External Chest Compressions

External chest compressions are required only if a pulse is not present. After each minute of rescue breathing, you should feel for a pulse. If a pulse cannot be felt, external chest compressions must be given.

If there is no pulse initially, external chest compressions must be given in addition to rescue breathing. This procedure is known as **cardiopulmonary resuscitation (CPR)**. External chest compressions require a smooth application of pressure over the lower half of the sternum. External pressure applied to the sternum causes pressure in the chest (intrathoracic) to increase, thus producing blood movement to the brain. Compressions must not be sharp or jabbing or applied over the tip of the sternum (xiphoid process). Proper hand position and placement on the child's chest are necessary to avoid internal injury such as bruising of the heart, laceration of the liver, or rupture of the spleen.

Blood flow in the carotid arteries as a result of external chest compressions is only one-fourth to one-third the normal flow, but it is adequate until advanced life support can be given. Because the blood circulates oxygen, chest compressions must be accompanied by rescue breathing.

Injuries are the leading cause of childhood deaths in the United States. During this century, trauma has replaced infectious disease as the most important threat to our children.

## Motor Vehicle

Motor vehicle-occupant injuries are a prominent cause of death for children of all ages. More than 200,000 children are treated in hospital emergency departments per year.

The highest death rates among preteenagers occur in the youngest children. Head injuries predominate as a cause of death.

The trauma causing most deaths and disabilities occurs a fraction of a second after a crash, when an unrestrained child strikes the vehicle interior. Proper use of car safety seats or seat belts will usually prevent injurious contact with the vehicle interior and keep the child from being ejected from the car. About one-tenth of children injured as motor vehicle occupants strike the vehicle interior during a sudden stop, turn, or swerve.

More than half of all deaths or severe injuries to motor vehicle occupants can be prevented by the use of restraints. In fact, properly used car safety seats for children appear to reduce the risk of severe injury or death in a crash by as much as 70 percent. Restraints of all types protect occupants by securing them to the vehicle so that their bodies stop more slowly in a crash and are less likely to be thrown against the vehicle's interior. Restraints also are designed to spread the impact forces widely over strong parts of the body.

Car safety seats should be used until a child outgrows them. Infant safety seats must be used facing the rear window so that frontal crash forces are spread across the infant's back. Misuse of seats is a common and important problem, because incorrectly used seats do not provide maximum protection and may even contribute to injury.

Passengers in the rear seat are better protected than passengers in the front seat in most crashes. Seat belts can be used to restrain a small child but are not as protective as safety seats.

## Pedestrians

Pedestrian injuries are the leading cause of death in children aged 4–8, with the peak at age 6. Although pedestrian fatalities to older children are often the result of "dart-outs" into traffic, fatalities to children younger than 5 tend to occur when a child is backed over in the home driveway by a vehicle driven by a parent.

The physical vulnerability of pedestrians is a major factor in their injury. A 50-pound child is no match for a 2,000- to 3,000-pound moving vehicle.

## Poisoning

Although poisoning is no longer a major cause of death in very young children, it remains a significant reason for hospitalizations and medical visits. The substances most commonly ingested are aspirin, solvents and petroleum products, tranquilizers, and iron compounds.

The reductions in poisoning deaths in young children are due to several factors, probably including the availability of poison-control centers, better emergency care, child-resistant packaging, reformulation of some poisonous substances such as lead paint, and reduced use of other substances such as kerosene.

## Animals

Every year, almost 2 percent of all children in the United States require hospital emergency room treatment because of an animal bite or sting, with dog bites being the most common source of injury. Infants have the highest death rate and are typically attacked by pet dogs in the home. The majority of fatally injured children aged one year or older had entered a fenced yard or wandered within reach of a chained dog.

Children aged 7–12 are at greatest risk of being bitten by dogs, primarily by their own dogs and by neighbors' dogs.

Male dogs have the highest rate of biting. Working and sporting dogs and certain breeds are especially likely to bite: german shepherds and collies have especially high rates of biting. Media and legislative attention has focused on pit bull terrier attacks, which are 42 percent of all U.S. fatalities in which the breed was known—several times more than any other breed.

## Firearms

Childhood shootings constitute a major public health problem. Many unintentional shootings occur when children mistake a loaded gun for a toy. Guns that are left loaded and unlocked in a home, kept there for protective purposes, too often result in family tragedy instead of family security.

## Definitions

**Cardiopulmonary resuscitation (CPR)** combines rescue breathing (also known as mouth-to-mouth breathing) and external chest compressions. *Cardio* refers to the heart, and *pulmonary* refers to the lungs. *Resuscitation* means "to revive." Proper and prompt CPR serves as a holding action by providing oxygen to the brain and heart until advanced cardiac life support can be provided.

**Basic life support (BLS)** refers to lifesaving procedures that focus on the victim's airway, breathing, and circulation. BLS includes rescue breathing, CPR, and obstructed airway management.

## Complications of CPR

The most common complication during CPR is fracture of the ribs, sternum, or clavicle because the rescuer's hands are misplaced. Bruises of the lungs and the heart surface can occur during improperly performed chest compressions. Broken ribs can puncture the lungs, liver, spleen, or heart. Rupture of the lungs can occur from excessive inflation of the lungs in children and in adults with chronic lung disease.

## When to Stop CPR

Continue CPR until one of the following occurs:

- The victim revives (regains pulse and breathing). Though revival is hoped for, most victims also require advanced cardiac procedures before ever regaining their heart and lung functions.
- You are replaced by either another trained rescuer or EMS personnel.
- A physician tells you to stop.
- You are too exhausted to continue.
- The scene becomes unsafe for you to continue.
- Cardiac arrest lasts longer than 30 minutes (with or without CPR, except in cases of severe hypothermia, according to the National Association of EMS Physicians).

Follow these steps to accomplish effective chest compression:

1. Place the child on his or her back on a firm, level surface. The lower extremities may be raised to promote the return of venous blood.

2. Locate the lower part of the child's sternum by sliding your middle and index fingers along the margin of the child's rib cage until the notch is located in the center of the lower chest where the ribs and the sternum meet. Keep the middle finger on the center of the notch and place your index finger on the lower end of the child's sternum, next to your middle finger.

3. Your fingers should be pointing away from you. After locating the tip of the sternum, lift your fingers and put the heel of the same hand immediately above where the index finger was. Extend your fingers but keep them off the child's chest wall to avoid rib fractures and other internal injuries. The heel of the hand must remain in contact with the chest during both the compression and the release to prevent bouncing or jerking movements.

4. Lean forward so your shoulder is directly over your hand. Keeping your arm straight, press straight downward on the sternum 1 to 1½ inches, using the weight of the upper part of your body, then relax pressure on the sternum completely. The pressure and relaxation phases of each chest compression should be of equal duration; do not pause between each phase. Be sure to give each compression straight downward. Pushing at an angle is less effective and creates pressure over the ends of the ribs where they attach to the sternum, resulting in injury to the victim. Keep the other hand on the child's forehead.

5. Give 5 chest compressions at a rate slightly faster than one every second. Perform each series of 5 compressions while counting aloud, "One, two, three, four, five," to achieve the rate of 100 compressions per minute.

6. After 5 compressions, immediately give one slow breath. After one breath, quickly reassess your hand location and position, then begin another cycle of 5 compressions and one breath.

7. After you have completed four cycles (which should take about one minute), check the child's pulse. If you cannot feel a pulse, continue CPR starting with 5 compressions. Check the pulse every few minutes.

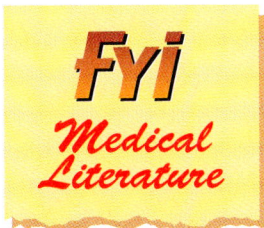

**Why Start with Chest Compressions?** After giving CPR and stopping to check the pulse, the rescuer should resume with chest compressions. The reason for this is that while the order does not appear to be important physiologically, a simple, consistent protocol—breathe, compress, breathe, compress—should be easier to learn and remember.

*Source:* American Heart Association, *Currents in Emergency Cardiac Care* 4(2):3 (Summer 1993).

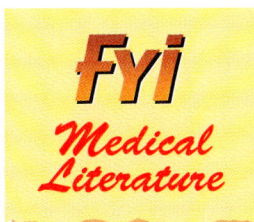

**Blows to the Chest Leading to Cardiac Arrest during Sports** A study was completed of twenty-five children and young adults 3 to 19 years of age who collapsed with cardiac arrest immediately after an unexpected blow to the chest, usually inflicted by an object such as a baseball or hockey puck. In each case, the impact to the chest was not judged to be extraordinary for the sport involved and did not appear to have sufficient force to cause death. Twelve victims collapsed instantaneously on impact, whereas thirteen remained conscious and physically active for a brief time before cardiac arrest. CPR was given within about 3 minutes to nineteen victims, but only two were revived.

*Source:* B. J. Maron et al., "Blunt Impact to the Chest Leading to Sudden Death from Cardiac Arrest during Sports Activities," *New England Journal of Medicine* 333(6):337–342 (August 1995).

## Historical Facts

Throughout the centuries, resuscitation attempts have included:

Unsuccessful methods

- slapping a victim
- dousing a victim with hot or cold water
- whipping a victim with stinging nettles
- making loud noises
- building a fire on a victim's abdomen

Occasionally successful methods

- rolling a drowned victim back and forth over a barrel
- throwing a victim across the back of a trotting horse
- blowing air into a victim with fireplace bellows

Sometimes successful methods

- pulling on a victim's arms
- pressing on a victim's back

The mouth-to-mouth breathing method (today known as rescue breathing) was sometimes reported prior to the 1950s. Since the 1950s, it has been the preferred method.

Medical researchers in 1960 discovered that compressing a victim's chest along with rescue breathing could help sustain life for a brief time period after breathing and pulse had stopped. At first, only physicians, nurses, and emergency medical aides were taught to perform the technique. In 1973, the American Heart Association declared CPR as a first aid procedure that should be taught to the public, not just to medically trained personnel.

The Heimlich maneuver (also known as abdominal thrusts) was first described by its developer, Dr. Henry J. Heimlich, in a 1974 medical journal.

**If you see a motionless child . . .**

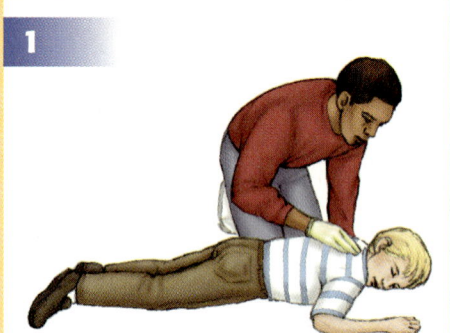

**1**

### Check responsiveness

- If spine injury is suspected, move child only if absolutely necessary.
- Tap child's shoulder.
- Shout near child's ear, "Are you okay?"

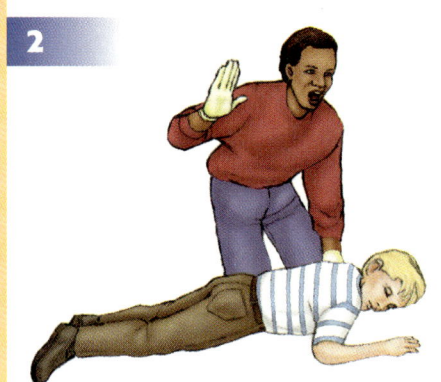

**2**

Send a bystander, if available, to activate the EMS. If you are alone, give rescue breathing or CPR for 1 minute before activating the EMS.

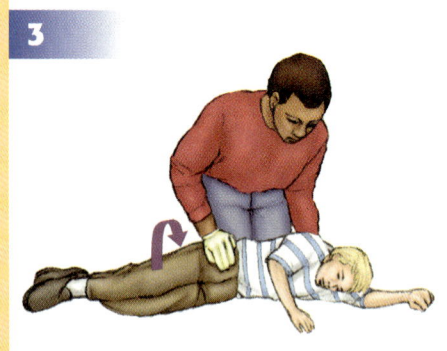

**3**

### Roll child onto back

- Gently roll child's head, body, and legs over at the same time. Do this without further injuring the child.

**4**

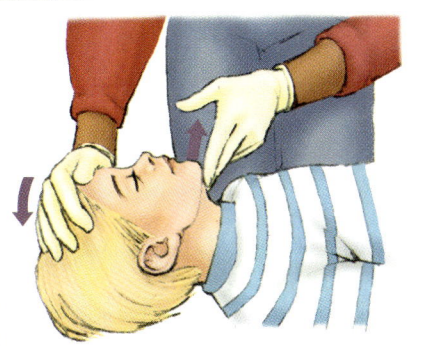

### Open airway (use head-tilt/chin-lift method)

- Place your hand nearest child's head on child's forehead and apply backward pressure to tilt head back.
- Place fingers of your other hand under bony part of jaw near chin and lift. Avoid pressing on soft tissues under jaw.
- Tilt head backward without closing child's mouth.
- Do *not* use your thumb to lift the chin.

### If you suspect a spine injury

Do *not* move child's head or neck. First try lifting chin without tilting head back. If breaths do not go in, slowly and gently bend the head back until breaths go in.

**5**

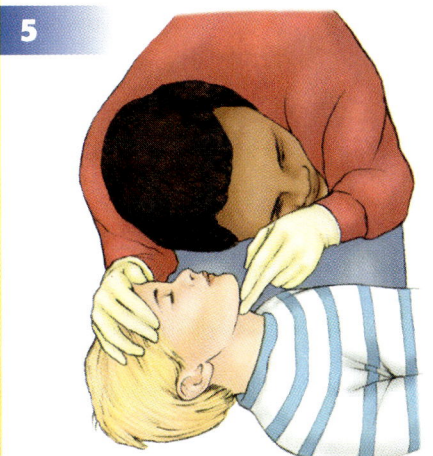

### Check for breathing (take 3–5 seconds)

- Place your ear over child's mouth and nose while keeping airway open.
- *Look* at child's chest to check for rise and fall; *listen* and *feel* for breathing.

**6**

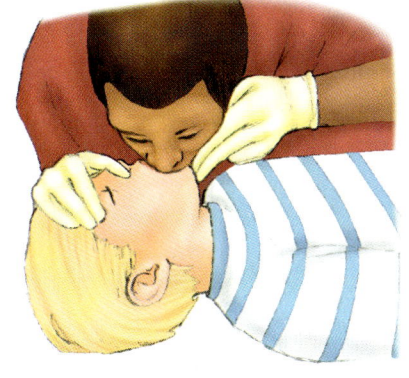

### Give 2 slow breaths

- Keep head tilted back with head-tilt/chin-lift to keep airway open.
- Pinch nose shut.
- Take a breath and seal your lips tightly around child's mouth.
- Give 2 slow breaths, each lasting 1 to 1½ seconds (you should take a breath after each breath given to victim).
- Watch chest rise to see if your breaths go in.
- Allow for chest deflation after each breath.

### If first breath did not go in

Retilt the head and try another breath. If second breath unsuccessful, suspect choking, also known as foreign body airway obstruction (use *Unconscious Child Foreign Body Airway Obstruction* procedures, described later in this section).

**7**

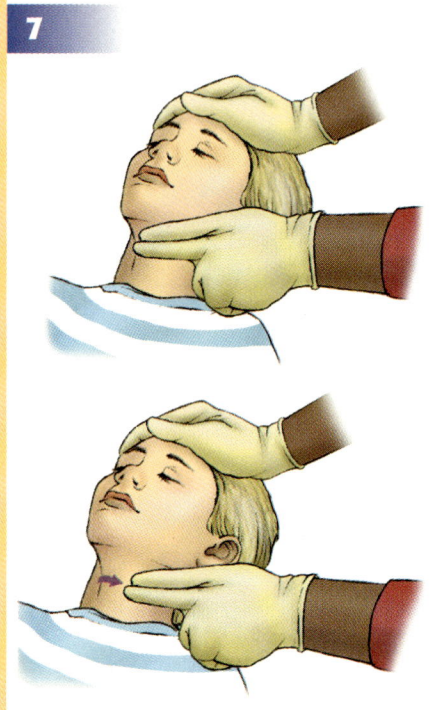

**Check for pulse** (5–10 seconds)

- Maintain head-tilt with your hand nearest the child's head on forehead.
- Locate Adam's apple with two fingers of hand nearest child's feet.
- Slide your fingers down into groove of neck on the side closest to you (do not use your thumb because you may feel your own pulse).
- Feel for carotid pulse (take 5–10 seconds). Carotid artery is used because it lies close to the heart and is accessible.

**8**

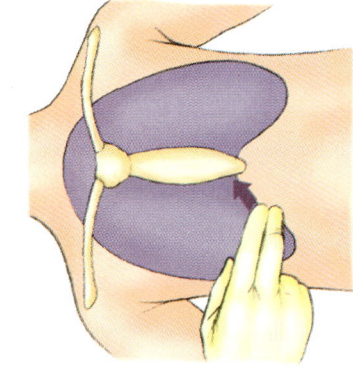

**Perform rescue procedures based upon what you found:**

**If there is a pulse but no breathing**

Give one rescue breath every 3 seconds. Use the same techniques for rescue breathing given in Step 6 but give only 1 breath. Every minute (20 breaths) stop and check the pulse to make sure there is a pulse. Continue until:

- Child starts breathing on his or her own.

OR

- Trained help, such as emergency medical technicians (EMTs), arrives and relieves you.

OR

- You are completely exhausted.

**If there is no pulse, give CPR**

- Find hand position.
    1. Slide the fingers of your hand nearest the child's feet up rib cage edge nearest to you to notch at the end of sternum.

**8**

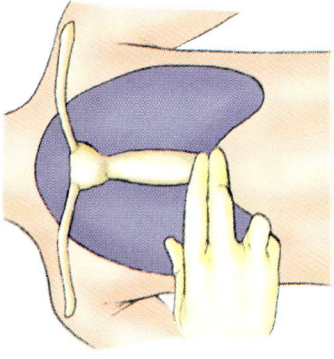

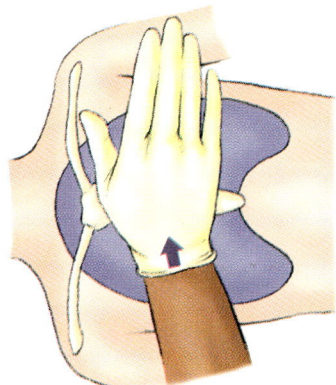

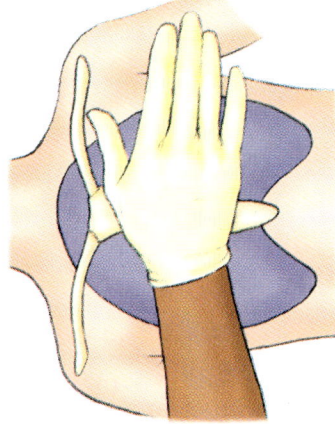

2. Place your middle finger on or in the notch and the index finger next to it.

3. Lift your fingers and hand off and put heel of the same hand on sternum immediately above where index finger was.

- Do 5 compressions.

1. Place your shoulder directly over your hand on the chest.

2. Keep the arm straight and elbow locked. Keep the other hand on the child's forehead to maintain head-tilt.

3. Push sternum straight down 1 to 1½ inches.

4. Do 5 compressions at a rate of 100 per minute. Count as you push down: "One, two, three, four, five."

5. Push smoothly; do not jerk or jab; do not stop at the top or at the bottom of the compression action.

6. When pushing, bend from your hips, not knees.

7. Keep fingers pointing across child's chest, away from you.

- Give 1 slow breath.

**9**

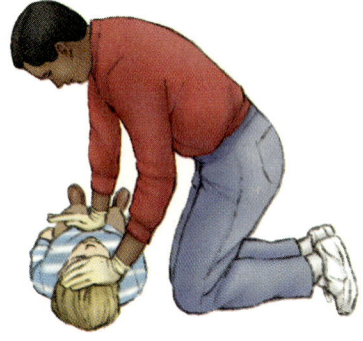

- Complete 19 more cycles in addition to the one above and recheck the pulse. *If there is no pulse,* restart CPR with chest compressions. Recheck the pulse every few minutes. *If there is a pulse,* give rescue breathing.

**10**

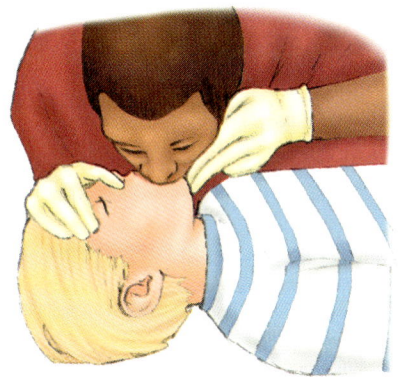

- Continue CPR or rescue breathing until:
  Child revives.
OR
  Trained help, such as emergency medical technicians (EMTs), arrives and relieves you.
OR
  You are completely exhausted.

# Airway Obstruction (Choking)

Children inhale all kinds of objects. Foods such as hot dogs, candy, peanuts, and grapes are major offenders because of their shape and consistencies. Non-food choking deaths are caused by balloons, balls and marbles, toys, and coins. Balloons are the top cause of non-food choking deaths in children.

## Recognizing Choking

Choking children vary as to whether the child (1) is conscious and has a partial airway obstruction, (2) is conscious and has a complete airway obstruction, (3) becomes unconscious as a result of complete airway obstruction, or (4) is found unconscious with complete airway obstruction.

A foreign body lodged in the airway may cause partial or complete airway obstruction. When a foreign body partially blocks the airway, either good or poor air exchange may result. When good air exchange is present, the child is able to make forceful coughing efforts in an attempt to relieve the obstruction. The child should be permitted and encouraged to cough. Sometimes, a good air exchange may progress to a poor air exchange.

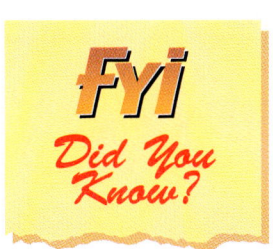

### Childhood Drownings

More than 2,000 children drown each year; in some states drowning is considered the leading cause of death for children under the age of 5. Many survivors of near-drowning have permanent neurologic disability. The two distinct high risk groups are children under 5 years and boys aged 15 to 19. Most drownings in the former group occur in residential pools. The outcome of an immersion is determined within a few minutes of the onset of immersion. This emphasizes the importance of prevention. Requiring pool fencing is the most promising strategy. Training in cardiopulmonary resuscitation is valuable.

*Source:* G. J. Wintemute, "Childhood Drowning and Near-Drowning in the United States," *American Journal of Diseases in Children* 144(6):663–669 (June 1990).

## Types of Upper Airway Obstruction

- *Tongue.* Unconsciousness produces relaxation of soft tissues, and the tongue can fall into the airway. "Swallowing one's tongue" is impossible, but the widespread belief that that can happen is explained by slippage of the relaxed tongue into the airway. The tongue is the most common cause of airway obstruction.
- *Foreign body.* The National Safety Council reports that 3,000 deaths occur in the United States each year because of foreign body airway obstruction. People, especially children, inhale all kinds of objects. Foods such as hot dogs, candy, peanuts, and grapes are major offenders because of their shapes and consistencies. Meat is the main cause of choking in adults. Balloons are the top cause of nonfood choking deaths in children, followed by balls, marbles, toys, and coins. Unconscious victims' airways also can be obstructed by a foreign body (e.g., vomit, teeth).
- *Swelling.* Severe allergic reactions (anaphylaxis) and irritants (e.g., smoke, chemicals) can cause swelling. Even a nonallergic person who is stung inside the throat by a bee, yellow jacket, or flying insect can experience swelling in the airway.
- *Spasm.* Water that is suddenly inhaled can cause a spasm in the throat. This happens in about 10 percent of all drownings. When such a spasm does not allow the lungs to fill with water, it is known as a "dry drowning."
- *Vomit.* Most people vomit when they are at or near death. Therefore, always expect vomit during CPR.

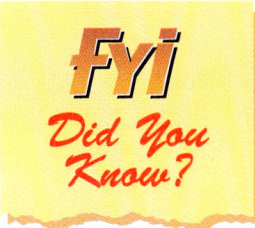

### Give CPR Early to Drowning Victim

An analysis of the records of 166 drowning victims from newborn to 14 years admitted to Los Angeles emergency departments indicates that children who receive mouth-to-mouth resuscitation or full CPR before EMS arrival "had significantly better neurological outcome" than children who did not receive immediate bystander care. About 75 percent of victims received immediate care; many caregivers had no formal training. After accounting for other variables, children who were revived without brain damage were 4.75 times more likely to have received resuscitative efforts.

The researchers recommended that CPR should be taught to all parents, siblings, and caretakers of children.

*Source:* D. N. Kyriacou et al., "Immediate Resuscitation Effect on Submersion Injury," *Pediatrics* 94(2):137–142 (August 1994).

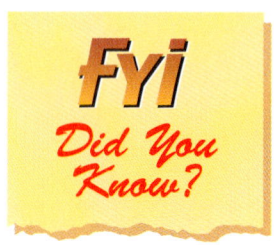

### Risk Factors for Drowning

A survey of 700 households showed deficits in knowledge of the importance of adult supervision and the recommended age at which to begin children's swimming instructions. Results showed a need for fencing that separates a swimming pool from a house and yard. Most reported that they did not know how to perform cardiopulmonary resuscitation (CPR) on an infant or child. More than 40 percent reported not knowing how to perform CPR on an adult.

*Source:* K. D. Liller et al., "Risk Factors for Drowning and Near-Drowning among Children in Hillsborough County, Florida," *Public Health Reports* 108(3):346–353 (May–June 1993).

A choking child who has poor air exchange has weak and ineffective coughs, and breathing becomes more difficult. The skin, the fingernail beds, and the inside of the mouth may appear bluish-gray in color (indicating **cyanosis**). Each attempt to inhale is usually accompanied by a high-pitched noise. A partial airway obstruction with poor air exchange should be treated as if it were a complete airway blockage.

Complete airway obstruction in a conscious child commonly occurs when the child has been eating. The child is unable to speak, breathe, or cough. When asked, "Can you speak?" the child is unable to respond verbally. Choking children with complete foreign body obstruction of the airway may instinctively reach up and clutch their necks to communicate that they are choking. This motion is known as the distress signal for choking. The child

becomes panicked and desperate and may appear pale in color. Because a complete obstruction prevents air from entering the lungs, oxygen deprivation occurs within a few minutes.

## Abdominal Thrusts

Giving abdominal thrusts to a choking child can dislodge the foreign body from the airway. To give abdominal thrusts to a choking child who is sitting or standing, position yourself behind the child. Place your arms around the child's waist and form a fist with one hand. Place the thumb side of the fist with the knuckles up against the child's abdomen slightly above the navel. With your other hand, grasp and hold your fist, then give up to five quick upward and inward thrusts to the child's abdomen. If the child is sitting in a chair, you probably will have to turn the child, since reaching around the child and the back of the chair usually is not practical.

To give abdominal thrusts to a child who is lying down, kneel and straddle the child's thighs. Place the heel of one hand against the child's abdomen slightly above the navel. Place the other hand over the first hand. Point the fingers of the bottom hand toward the child's head. Then give five quick inward, upward thrusts. Use this method, too, if you are unable to reach around the waist of a conscious child.

## Finger Sweep of the Mouth

Use this maneuver only if the child is unconscious and you can see the foreign object. Do *not* perform blind finger sweeps.

First, open the child's mouth by means of the tongue-jaw lift. With the child's head up, place your thumb in the child's mouth over the tongue. Then grasp the child's tongue and lower jaw between your thumb and fingers and lift upward.

If you are unable to open the child's mouth, use the crossed-finger technique. To perform that maneuver, cross your index finger and thumb and use them as a wedge to push the child's teeth apart. Once the mouth is opened, insert a thumb for the tongue-jaw lift.

While keeping the child's mouth open with the tongue-jaw lift, use the index finger of your other hand to sweep down along the inside of one cheek. This finger should probe deeply into the throat to the base of the tongue. Using a hooking action, try to dislodge the foreign body and maneuver it so it can be removed. Be careful not to force the object deeper into the airway.

## Conscious Choking Children

First determine if the child has good or poor air exchange. A child with good air exchange is able to speak, cough forcefully, and make effective breathing efforts. Encourage such a child to cough; do not interfere with the child's efforts to expel the object.

For a conscious child with a partial airway obstruction who has poor air exchange, help the child as for a complete obstruction. Poor air exchange is marked by ineffective, weak coughing, high-pitched noise, breathing difficulty, possible cyanosis, and inability to speak. To assist these children:

1. Ask, "Can you speak?"
2. If the child is unable to speak, give five abdominal thrusts.
3. Assess the child and your technique.
4. Repeat the sequence of five thrusts and a reassessment until the airway is clear or the child becomes unconscious.

## Unconscious Choking Children

To help an unconscious choking child:

1. Determine the child's responsiveness.
2. Call for help—either send someone or call yourself.
3. Open the child's airway using the head-tilt/chin-lift method.
4. Determine if the child is breathing by looking at the chest and listening for air coming out of the mouth and nose.
5. Give two slow breaths. If the first breath does not go in, retilt the child's head and try a second breath. *The breaths not going in indicates choking.*
6. Give five abdominal thrusts.
7. Using one hand, open the child's mouth with the tongue-jaw lift. If you can see the foreign object, use your index finger to sweep the mouth and remove it.
8. Reposition the child in a head-tilt/chin-lift position and give one breath.
9. If unsuccessful, repeat the sequence of five thrusts, mouth check, one breath until the airway is clear or until the child becomes conscious.

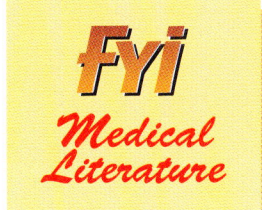

### Why No Blind Finger Sweeps in Children?

The blind finger sweep technique presents a significant risk for infants and children that is not a factor for adult victims. Given the small size of the infant's and child's upper airway, the rescuer's fingers may inadvertently push the object farther down into the airway during a blind finger sweep. This is less likely in the adult victim because of the increased length of the upper airway. Therefore, for infants and small children, a finger sweep is recommended only when the object is visible.

*Source:* American Heart Association, *Currents in Emergency Cardiac Care* 6(1):9 (Spring 1995).

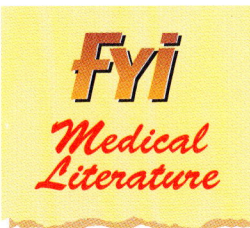

### Should Abdominal Thrusts Be Used for Near-Drowning?

The Institute of Medicine committee of the National Academy of Sciences recommendations on using abdominal thrusts on drowning victims:

- There is *no evidence* that death from drowning is frequently caused by aspiration of a solid foreign body.
- The *evidence is insufficient* that an abdominal thrust is useful for the removal of aspirated liquid.
- There is *no evidence* that substantial amounts of water are aspirated by near-drowning victims or that such aspirated liquid causes brain damage and death.
- The *evidence does not support* routine use of abdominal thrusts in the care of near-drowning victims.

The committee had concerns about routine use of abdominal thrusts for treatment of near-drowning because of the time delay the maneuver would cause, possible complications of the maneuver, especially if cervical fracture is present, and the difficulty of teaching a protocol for CPR in the near-drowning victim that differs from CPR protocols for all other victims.

*Source:* American Heart Association, *Currents in Emergency Cardiac Care* 6(2):8 (Summer 1995).

# Conscious Child Foreign Body Airway Obstruction (Choking)

**If child is conscious and cannot speak, breathe, or cough . . .**

**1**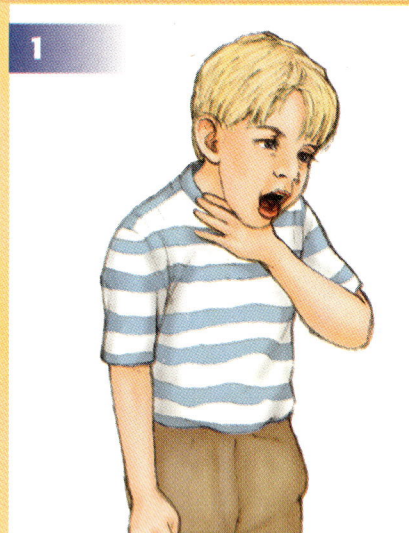

**Give up to 5 abdominal thrusts** (Heimlich maneuver)

- Kneel or stand behind the child.
- Wrap your arms around child's waist. (Do not allow your forearms to touch the ribs.)
- Make a fist with one hand and place the thumb side just above child's navel and well below the tip of the sternum.
- Grasp fist with your other hand.
- Press fist into child's abdomen with 5 quick upward thrusts.
- Each thrust should be a separate and distinct effort to dislodge the object.

After every 5 abdominal thrusts, check the child and your technique.

**2**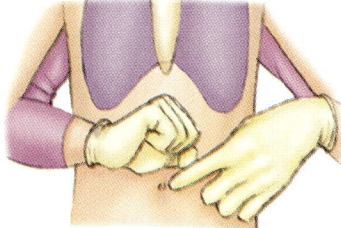

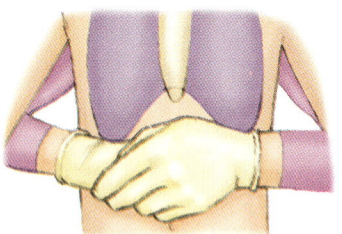

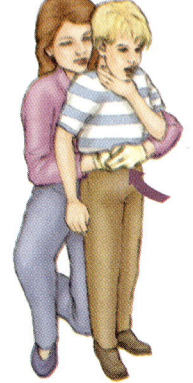

**Repeat cycles of up to 5 abdominal thrusts until**

- Child coughs up object.

OR

- Child starts to breathe or coughs forcefully.

OR

- Child becomes unconscious (activate EMS and start methods for an unconscious child, visually checking the mouth for a foreign object first).

OR

- You are relieved by EMS or other trained person.

Reassess child and your technique after every 5 thrusts.

# Unconscious Child Foreign Body Airway Obstruction (Choking)

**If child is unconscious, you gave 1 breath that did not go in, retilted the child's head and gave a second breath that did not go in . . .**

**1**

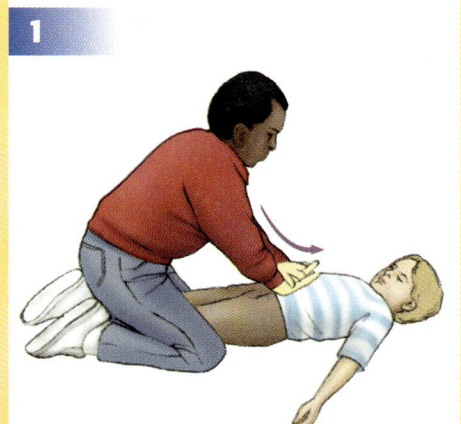

**Give up to 5 abdominal thrusts** (Heimlich maneuver)

- Kneel at child's feet or straddle child's thighs.
- Put heel of one hand against middle of child's abdomen slightly above navel and well below sternum's notch (fingers of hand should point toward child's head).
- Put other hand directly on top of first hand.
- Press inward and upward using both hands with up to 5 quick abdominal thrusts.
- Each thrust should be distinct and a real attempt made to relieve the airway obstruction. Keep heel of hand in contact with abdomen between abdominal thrusts.

**2**

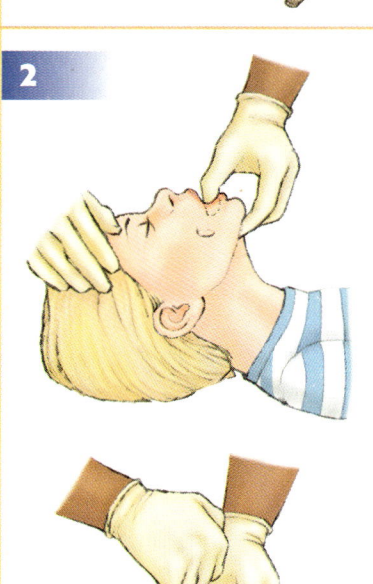

**Check mouth for foreign object**

Perform finger sweep only if you can see foreign body: DO NOT perform a blind finger sweep.

- Use your thumb and fingers to grasp child's jaw and tongue and lift upward to pull tongue away from back of throat.
- If you can see foreign body, using index or little finger of your other hand, slide finger down along the inside of one cheek deeply into mouth and use a hooking action across to other cheek to remove foreign object.

**3**

**If Steps 1 and 2 are unsuccessful**

Cycle through the following steps in rapid sequence until the object is expelled or EMS arrives:

- Give 1 rescue breath.
- Do up to 5 abdominal thrusts.
- Look into the mouth; if you can see foreign body, remove it with finger sweep.

# Child Basic Life Support Proficiency Checklist

## Child Rescue Breathing

|  | S | P | I |
|---|---|---|---|
| 1. Check responsiveness. | ☐ | ☐ | ☐ |
| 2. Send a bystander, if available, to call EMS. | ☐ | ☐ | ☐ |
| 3. Roll child onto back. | ☐ | ☐ | ☐ |
| 4. Airway open. | ☐ | ☐ | ☐ |
| 5. Breathing check. | ☐ | ☐ | ☐ |
| 6. 2 slow breaths. | ☐ | ☐ | ☐ |
| 7. Check pulse at carotid. | ☐ | ☐ | ☐ |
| 8. Rescue breathing (1 every 3 seconds). | ☐ | ☐ | ☐ |
| 9. If alone, call EMS after 1 minute. | ☐ | ☐ | ☐ |
| 10. Recheck pulse and breathing after first minute, then every few minutes. | ☐ | ☐ | ☐ |

## Child One-Rescuer CPR

|  | S | P | I |
|---|---|---|---|
| 1. Check responsiveness. | ☐ | ☐ | ☐ |
| 2. Send a bystander, if available, to call EMS. | ☐ | ☐ | ☐ |
| 3. Roll child onto back. | ☐ | ☐ | ☐ |
| 4. Airway open. | ☐ | ☐ | ☐ |
| 5. Breathing check. | ☐ | ☐ | ☐ |
| 6. 2 slow breaths. | ☐ | ☐ | ☐ |
| 7. Check pulse at carotid. | ☐ | ☐ | ☐ |
| 8. Hand position using same hand used to locate tip of sternum. | ☐ | ☐ | ☐ |
| 9. 5 compressions with only 1 hand. | ☐ | ☐ | ☐ |
| 10. 1 slow breath. | ☐ | ☐ | ☐ |
| 11. Continue CPR for 1 minute (19 more cycles, for total of 20). | ☐ | ☐ | ☐ |

## (Child One-Rescuer CPR continued)

|  | S | P | I |
|---|---|---|---|
| 12. If alone, call EMS after 1 minute. | ☐ | ☐ | ☐ |
| 13. Recheck pulse. | ☐ | ☐ | ☐ |
| 14. Continue CPR (start with compressions). | ☐ | ☐ | ☐ |
| 15. Recheck pulse after first minute, then every few minutes. | ☐ | ☐ | ☐ |

## Conscious Child Choking Management

|  | S | P | I |
|---|---|---|---|
| 1. Recognize choking. | ☐ | ☐ | ☐ |
| 2. Up to 5 abdominal thrusts. | ☐ | ☐ | ☐ |
| 3. Reassess. | ☐ | ☐ | ☐ |
| 4. Repeat cycles of up to 5 thrusts; reassess after each cycle. | ☐ | ☐ | ☐ |

## Unconscious Child Choking Management

|  | S | P | I |
|---|---|---|---|
| 1. Check responsiveness. | ☐ | ☐ | ☐ |
| 2. Send a bystander, if available, to call EMS. | ☐ | ☐ | ☐ |
| 3. Roll child onto back. | ☐ | ☐ | ☐ |
| 4. Airway open. | ☐ | ☐ | ☐ |
| 5. Breathing check. | ☐ | ☐ | ☐ |
| 6. Try 2 slow breaths. (If first breath unsuccessful, retilt head and try 1 more breath.) | ☐ | ☐ | ☐ |
| 7. Up to 5 abdominal thrusts. | ☐ | ☐ | ☐ |
| 8. Check mouth for foreign object (finger sweep only if object is visible). | ☐ | ☐ | ☐ |
| 9. Try 1 slow breath. | ☐ | ☐ | ☐ |
| 10. Repeat sequence of 5 thrusts, mouth check, 1 breath. | ☐ | ☐ | ☐ |

# CPR Review

| Action | Infant (0–1 year) | Child (1–8 years) |
| --- | --- | --- |
| **How to open airway?** | Head-tilt/chin-lift | Head-tilt/chin-lift |
| **How to check breathing?** | Look at chest and listen and feel for air (3–5 seconds). | Look at chest and listen and feel for air (3–5 seconds). |
| **What kinds of breaths?** | Slow, make chest rise and fall | Slow, make chest rise and fall |
| **Where to check pulse?** | Brachial artery (5–10 seconds) | Carotid artery (5–10 seconds) |
| **Hand position for chest compressions?** | 1 finger's width below imaginary line between nipples | 1 finger's width above tip of sternum |
| **Compress with?** | 2 fingers | Heel of 1 hand |
| **Compression depth?** | ½–1 inch | 1–1½ inches |
| **Compression rate?** | 100 per minute | 100 per minute |
| **Compression:breath ratio?** | 5:1 | 5:1 |
| **How to count for compression rate?** | 1, 2, 3, 4, 5, breathe | 1, 2, 3, 4, 5, breathe |
| **How often to reassess?** | After the first minute, then every few minutes | After the first minute, then every few minutes |
| **After reassessment, resume CPR with?** | Compressions | Compressions |
| **How often to give only breaths during rescue breathing?** | Every 3 seconds | Every 3 seconds |

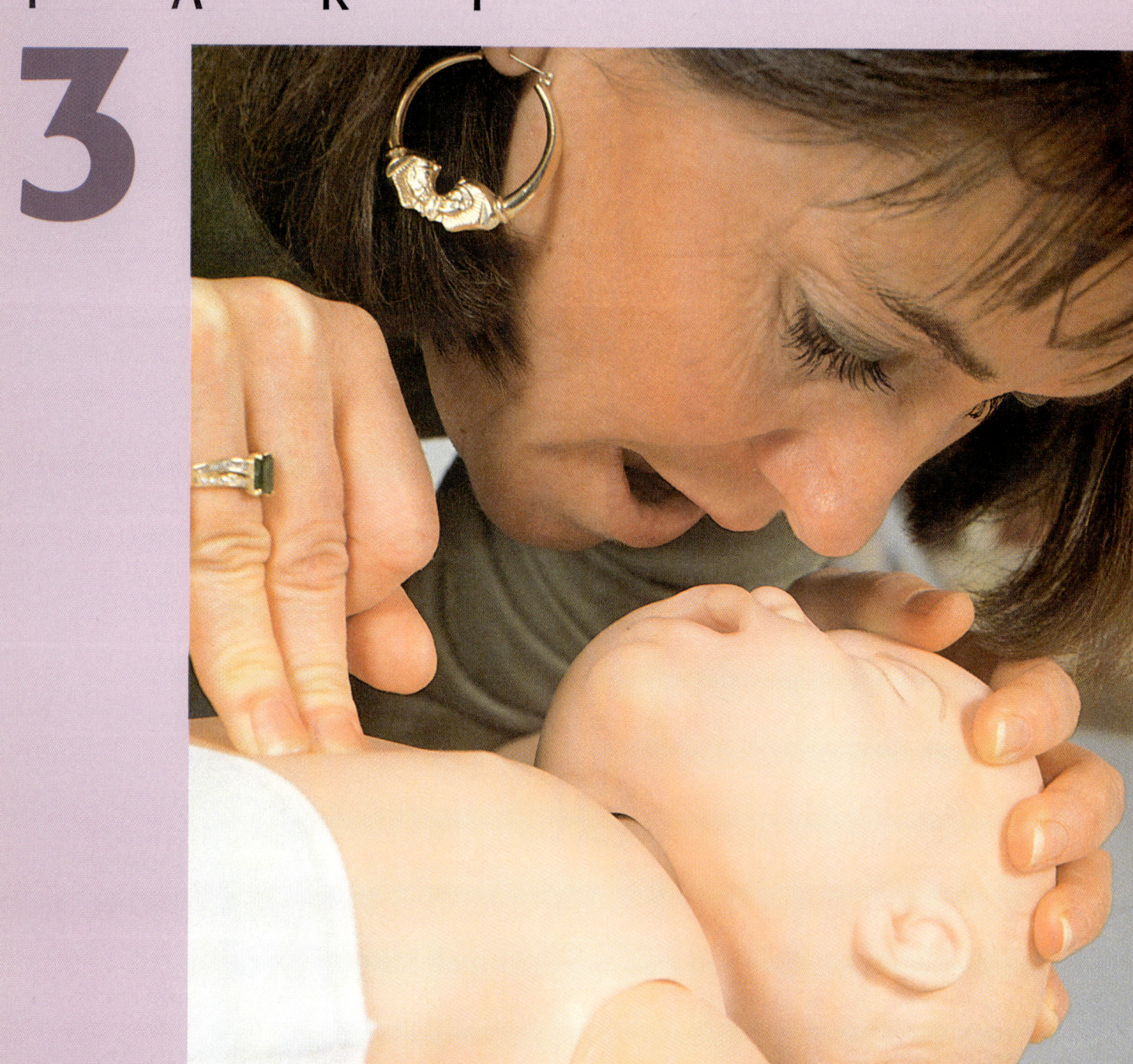

# INFANT BASIC LIFE SUPPORT*

Basic life support techniques for an infant (under one year) differ from those for an adult or child. Initially occurring cardiac arrest in infants is rare. Usually, infants have a respiratory arrest with cardiac arrest developing later because the heart muscle did not receive sufficient oxygen.

## Infant Rescue Breathing and CPR

### Check Responsiveness

The first priority in a cardiopulmonary emergency is to determine the infant's responsiveness. This is done by tapping the infant and speaking loudly. If basic life support is necessary, give resuscitation for one minute before activating the EMS. The rescuer should shout for help if alone.

### Positioning an Unresponsive Infant

Properly position the infant so that if any resuscitation efforts are needed, they can be performed. If the infant is found lying facedown, turn the infant as a complete unit onto his or her back. The infant's head and neck should always be supported with one of your hands so that they remain aligned with the rest of the body and do not twist.

### Opening the Airway

After unresponsiveness has been determined and the infant has been properly positioned, open the airway by using the head-tilt/chin-lift method. To do this, place one hand to apply pressure on the infant's forehead to gently tilt the head backward. Do not overtilt the head backward because it can block the airway because of the pliability of the infant's tissues. To lift the chin, place the finger(s) of your other hand under the bony part of the jaw. Then lift your fingers to bring the chin up. The fingers should not press on the soft tissue under the infant's chin because it can interfere with the opening of the airway. While the chin is lifted, the hand on the forehead maintains the head-tilt position of the infant. Sometimes, opening the airway may be all that is necessary for the infant to breathe.

*Based on the American Heart Association, Guidelines for Cardiopulmonary Resuscitation and Emergency Cardiac Care, *JAMA* 268:2172 (1992).

When a spine injury is suspected, open the airway using the chin-lift without tilting the head back. If the airway remains blocked, tilt the head slowly and gently until the airway is open. Another technique for a suspected spine-injured infant is using a jaw thrust without a head tilt. While stabilizing the head, place the fingers of each hand behind the angles of the infant's lower jaw on each side of the head and move the lower jaw forward without tilting the head backward; however, it may be necessary to tilt the head slightly if the airway cannot be opened.

## Check for Breathing

After unresponsiveness has been determined and the airway has been opened, you should look, listen, and feel for breathing. You should (1) look to see whether there is any visible movement of the infant's chest, (2) listen for air by placing your ear next to the infant's mouth and nose, and (3) feel for air by placing your cheek next to the infant's mouth and nose. If breathing is present, you will see the infant's chest rise and fall, hear air coming from the infant's mouth and nose, and feel air against your own cheek.

## Rescue Breathing

To give rescue breaths to an infant, place your mouth over the infant's nose and mouth, forming an airtight seal. Give two slow breaths, taking time to quickly breathe between them.

If both breaths went into the infant, check the pulse. If the first breath did not go in, retilt the infant's head and try a second breath.

The breaths for an infant should be limited to the amount needed to raise the chest. For infants, use shallow puffs of air.

To perform rescue breathing for an infant, follow these steps:

1. Make sure the infant's head is positioned with a moderate head-tilt/chin-lift to open the airway.

2. Form an airtight seal over the infant's nose and mouth.

3. Give two breaths using shallow puffs of air.

4. Watch to see if the infant's chest rises.

5. Remove your mouth to allow the air to come out and move your head away as you take another breath.

If the first breath did not go in, retilt the infant's head and try a second breath. If breaths do not go

### Basic Life Support Steps for a Child or Infant Victim

**E:** **E**stablish unresponsiveness.
**S:** **S**end bystander, if available, to activate EMS (usually call 911).
**P:** **P**osition victim on back.

**A:** **A**irway open. Use head-tilt/chin-lift or jaw thrust.
**B:** **B**reathing check. Look, listen, and feel for 3–5 seconds.
  • If victim is breathing and spine injury is not suspected, place victim in recovery position.
  • If victim is not breathing, give 2 slow breaths; watch chest rise.
    - If 2 breaths go in, proceed to step C.
    - If first breath did not go in, retilt head and try 1 more breath.
    - If second breath did not go in, then . . .
    *For a child:* Give 5 abdominal thrusts; perform tongue-jaw lift and if object is seen perform a finger sweep; give 1 breath. Repeat sequence of 5 thrusts, mouth check, 1 breath.
    *For an infant:* Give 5 back blows and 5 chest thrusts; perform tongue-jaw lift and if object is seen perform a finger sweep; give 1 breath. Repeat sequence of 5 blows, 5 thrusts, mouth check, 1 breath.
**C:** **C**irculation check (for 5–10 seconds).
  • *For a child:* Check carotid pulse.
  • *For an infant:* Check brachial pulse.
  • If there is a pulse but no breathing, give rescue breathing (1 breath every 3 seconds).
  • If no pulse, give CPR (cycles of 5 chest compressions followed by 1 breath).
After 1 minute (20 cycles of CPR or 20 breaths of rescue breathing), check pulse.
  • If you are alone, activate EMS.
  • If there is no pulse, give CPR (cycles of 5 compressions and 1 breath) starting with chest compressions.
  • If there is a pulse but no breathing, give rescue breathing.

in, see the section on unconscious choking management on pages 46 and 49.

If the breaths went in and the infant has a pulse, continue giving rescue breathing. Because infants breathe faster than adults, breathe into an infant once every three seconds or 20 times a minute. Between breaths, remove your mouth from the infant's to allow air to flow out of the infant's lungs. As you remove your mouth, you should turn your head to the side to see if the infant's chest fell after each breath. For rescue breathing, breathe into the infant for the first second, count "one–one thousand," then take a breath yourself for the third second.

**Gastric Distention**    Rescue breaths tend to cause stomach or gastric distention more often in infants than in adults. Minimize this problem by limiting the breaths to the amount needed to make the chest rise. Avoid overinflating the lungs. Gastric distention can cause regurgitation and aspiration of stomach contents.

## Check for Pulse

After a nonbreathing infant has been given two breaths, the pulse must be checked. For an infant, the brachial pulse is used. An infant's neck is short and chubby, which makes it difficult to feel the carotid pulse. The brachial pulse can be found on the inside of the upper arm midway between the armpit and elbow. Feeling for the brachial pulse in an infant requires the use of the index and middle fingers of one hand. Place your thumb on the outside of the infant's arm midway between the shoulder and elbow. Place the tips of your index and middle fingers on the inside of the infant's arm opposite your thumb. The thumb is used to help with hand placement only, not to feel for the infant's pulse. Light pressure is applied toward the underlying bone to feel for the pulse. While checking the brachial pulse, keep your other hand on the infant's forehead to maintain the head-tilt position.

Should a pulse exist but breathing is absent, continue rescue breathing. A rescue breath is given once every three seconds or 20 times a minute. After 20 breaths, you should activate the EMS.

## Chest Compressions

An infant without a pulse requires both rescue breathing and external chest compressions. The proper chest compression point in an infant is the midsternum. To locate this area, imagine a line connecting the infant's nipples. Place three fingers (index, middle, and ring) with the index finger next to the imaginary nipple line on the infant's feet side. Lift the index finger off the chest.

Use the two remaining fingers to apply the chest compressions. Press the infant's midsternum

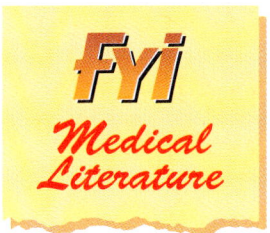

## Reasons for Certain Techniques

### Early EMS Access

Unlike rescuers of adults, rescuers of children and infants should provide about one minute of basic life support before activating the emergency medical service (EMS). To keep suggested numbers easy to recall, rescuers should provide rescue breathing for 20 breaths or perform 20 cycles of five compressions and one ventilation before activating the EMS. The number 20 was selected to enable consistency between the number of breaths and the number of compression/breathing cycles performed before activation of the EMS. Although 20 cycles of compressions and ventilation may take slightly longer than one minute, this represents a sufficiently close approximation.

### Rescue Breathing

If breathing is absent but a pulse is present, rescue breathing should be provided at a rate of 20 breaths per minute (about 1 breath every 3 seconds) for an infant or child. After about one minute of rescue breathing, the EMS should be activated.

### Compression Rate

In order to simplify the BLS guidelines, the compression rates for children and infants are identical—100 per minute for children and at least 100 per minute for infants. With pauses for breathing, the actual number of compressions provided is at least 80 per minute.

### Hand Placement

Using one hand to maintain head position during chest compressions minimizes the time required to open the airway and provide breathing.

*Source:* American Heart Association, *Currents in Emergency Cardiac Care* 3(4):20 (Winter 1992).

(area between the nipples) one-half to one inch with the middle and ring finger. Either place your other hand under the infant's shoulder to provide support or keep it on the infant's forehead to keep the head tilted. If the infant is carried during CPR, the length of the body is on the rescuer's forearm with the head kept level with the trunk.

An infant's heart rate is faster than an adult's and so the rate of compressions must also be faster. The infant compression rate is 100 per minute. External chest compressions must always be com-

## Airway Obstruction

- Partial airway obstruction (child or infant is alert and sitting):
  - High-pitched inhalation sound, crowing, or noisy breathing
  - Child is responsive
  - First aid: Allow position of comfort; assist young child to sit up (may sit on parent's lap); do not lay child or infant down
- Complete airway obstruction and altered mental status or cyanosis (blue skin color) and partial obstruction:
  - No crying or speaking and cyanosis
    a. Child's cough becomes ineffective
    b. Increased breathing difficulty accompanied by high-pitched inhalation sound
    c. Child or infant becomes unresponsive
    d. Altered mental status
  - First aid: Clear airway using either child foreign body obstruction procedures or infant foreign body obstruction procedures
- Attempt rescue breathing

## Breathing Emergencies

- Breathing distress precedes respiratory failure and is indicated by any of the following:
  - Breathing rate >60 in infants
  - Breathing rate >30–40 in children
  - Nasal flaring
  - High-pitched inhalation sound
  - Cyanosis (blue skin color)
  - Altered mental status (e.g., combative, unresponsive)
- Respiratory failure/arrest:
  - Breathing rate <10 per minute in child
  - Breathing rate <20 per minute in infant
  - Unresponsive
  - No pulse

## Sudden Infant Death Syndrome (SIDS)

- Signs and symptoms:
  - Sudden death in the first year of life
  - Causes are not clearly understood
  - Baby is most commonly discovered in the early morning
- First aid:
  - Complete ABC assessment
  - Comfort, calm, and reassure the parents while awaiting EMS
    a. Try to resuscitate unless the baby is stiff
    b. Parents will be in agony from emotional distress, remorse, and guilt; avoid any comments that might suggest blame

## Child Abuse

- Physical abuse and neglect are the two forms of child abuse:
  - Abuse: improper or excessive action so as to injure or cause harm
  - Neglect: giving insufficient attention or respect to someone who has a claim to that attention
- Signs and symptoms of abuse:
  - Multiple bruises in various stages of healing
  - Patterns of injury (e.g., cigarette burns, whip marks, hand prints)
  - Fresh burns such as scalding, untreated burns, body part dipped
  - Parents seem inappropriately unconcerned
  - Conflicting explanations of injury
- Signs and symptoms of neglect:
  - Lack of adult supervision
  - Malnourished-appearing child
  - Unsafe living environment
  - Untreated soft tissue injuries
- Do not accuse parents or guardians
- State law requires reporting:
  - Report what you see and what you hear
  - Do not comment on what you think

bined with rescue breathing. The ratio of compressions to breaths is 5 to 1. Each series of five compressions is performed while the rescuer says aloud "One, two, three, four, five." After the fifth compression, the rescuer opens the infant's airway and gives one breath.

After the first minute of CPR, and if a second rescuer is not available, activate the EMS. Every few minutes feel the pulse.

The procedures for performing rescue breathing and external chest compressions on an infant are as follows:

1. Determine responsiveness by tapping the infant; if the infant is lying facedown, turn him or her onto their back.
2. Make sure the infant's head is positioned with a moderate head-tilt/chin-lift to open the airway.

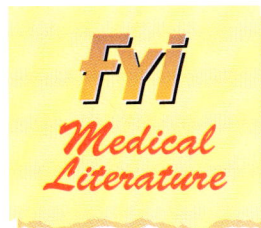

## Facts about Sudden Infant Death Syndrome (SIDS)

Many more children die of SIDS in a year than all who die of cancer, heart disease, pneumonia, child abuse, AIDS, cystic fibrosis, and muscular dystrophy combined . . .

### What Is SIDS?

- Sudden Infant Death Syndrome (SIDS) is a medical term that describes the sudden death of an infant that remains unexplained after all known and possible causes have been carefully ruled out through autopsy, death scene investigation, and review of the medical history. SIDS is responsible for more deaths than any other cause in childhood for babies one month to one year of age, claiming 150,000 victims in the United States in this generation alone—7,000 babies each year—*nearly one baby every hour of every day.* It strikes families of all races, ethnic, and socioeconomic origins without warning; neither parent nor physician can predict that something is going wrong. In fact, most SIDS victims appear healthy prior to death.

### What Causes SIDS?

- While there are still no adequate medical explanations for SIDS deaths, current theories include: (1) stress in a normal baby, caused by infection or other factors; (2) a birth defect; (3) failure to develop; and/or (4) a critical period when all babies are especially vulnerable, such as a time of rapid growth.

- Many new studies have been launched to learn how and why SIDS occurs. Scientists are exploring the development and function of the nervous system, the brain, the heart, breathing and sleep patterns, body chemical balances, autopsy findings, and environmental factors. It is likely that SIDS, like many other medical disorders, will eventually have more than one explanation.

### Can SIDS Be Prevented?

- No, not yet. But, some recent studies have begun to isolate several risk factors that, though not causes of SIDS in and of themselves, may play a role in some cases. (*It is important that, since the causes of SIDS remain unknown, SIDS parents refrain from concluding that their child care practices may have caused their baby's death.*)

### Some Basic Facts about SIDS:

- SIDS is a definite medical entity and is the major cause of death in infants after the first month of life.
- SIDS claims the lives of over 7,000 American babies each year . . . *nearly one baby every hour of every day.*
- SIDS victims appear to be healthy prior to death.
- Currently, SIDS cannot be predicted or prevented, even by a physician.
- There appears to be no suffering; death occurs very rapidly, usually during sleep.

### What SIDS Is Not:

- SIDS is **not** caused by external suffocation.
- SIDS is **not** caused by vomiting and choking.
- SIDS is **not** contagious.
- SIDS does **not** cause pain or suffering in the infant.
- SIDS can**not** be predicted.

*Source:* SIDS Network. Used with permission.

---

3. Check for breathing.
4. If breathing is absent, form an airtight seal over the infant's nose and mouth, and give two breaths using shallow puffs of air; watch to see if the infant's chest rises. Remove your mouth to allow the air to come out and move your head away as you take another breath. If the first breath did not go in, retilt the infant's head and try a second breath. If breaths do not go in, see the section on unconscious choking management on pages 46 and 49.
5. Check for a pulse at the brachial pulse point. If the breaths went in and the infant has a pulse, continue giving rescue breathing. Because infants breathe faster than adults, breathe into an infant once every three seconds or 20 times a minute. Between breaths, remove your mouth from the infant's to allow air to flow out of the

**If you see a motionless infant . . .**

**1**

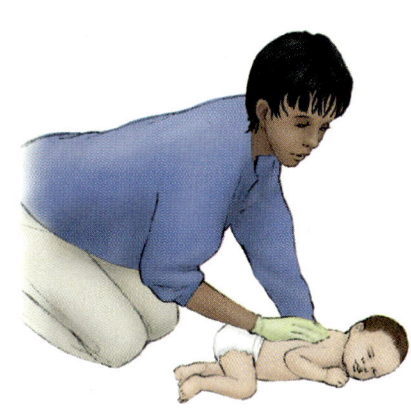

**Check responsiveness**
- If spine injury is suspected, move only if absolutely necessary.
- Tap infant's shoulder.

**2**

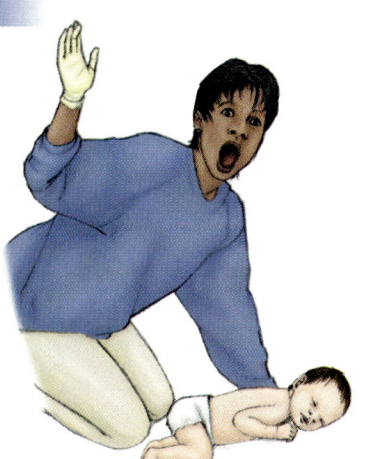

**Send bystander, if available, to activate EMS. If you are alone, give rescue breathing or CPR for 1 minute before activating EMS.**

**3**

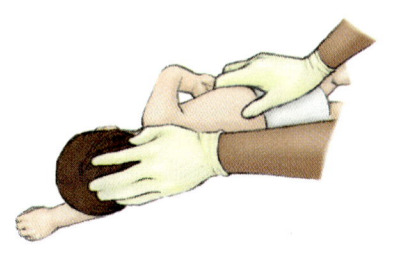

**Roll infant onto back**
Gently roll infant's head, body, and legs over at the same time (avoid twisting).

**4**

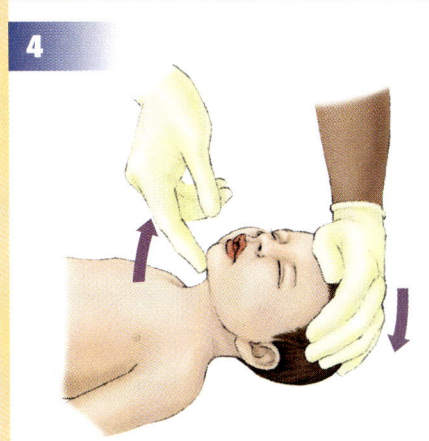

**Open airway** (use head-tilt/chin-lift method)

- Place your hand nearest infant's head on infant's forehead and apply backward pressure to tilt head back (known as the "sniffing" or neutral position).
- Place fingers of other hand under bony part of jaw near chin and lift. Avoid pressing on soft tissues under jaw.
- Tilt head backward without closing infant's mouth.
- Do not use your thumb to lift the chin.

**If you suspect a spine injury**

Do not move infant's head or neck. First try lifting chin without tilting head back. If breaths do not go in, slowly and gently bend the head back until breaths can go in.

**5**

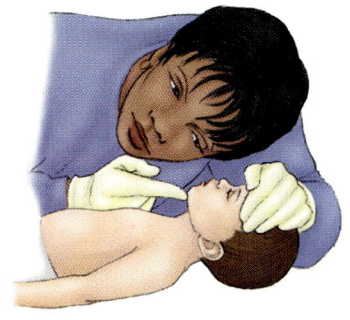

**Check for breathing** (take 3–5 seconds)

- Place your ear over infant's mouth and nose while keeping airway open.
- Look at infant's chest to check for rise and fall; listen and feel for breathing.

**6**

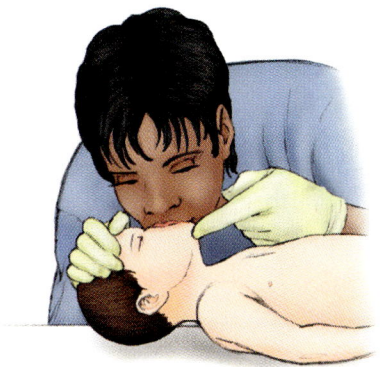

**Give 2 slow breaths**

- Keep head tilted back with head-tilt/chin-lift to keep airway open.
- With your mouth make a seal over infant's mouth and nose.
- Give 2 slow breaths, each lasting 1 to 1½ seconds (you should take a breath after each breath given).
- Watch chest rise to see if your breaths go in.
- Allow for chest deflation after each breath.

**If first breath did not go in**

Retilt the head and try another breath. If second breath is unsuccessful, suspect choking, also known as foreign body airway obstruction (refer to the *Unconscious Infant with Foreign Body Airway Obstruction (Choking)* section).

**7**

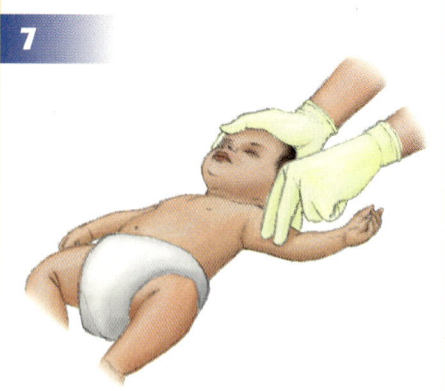

### Check for pulse

- Maintain head tilt with hand nearest head on forehead.
- Feel for pulse on the inside of the upper arm between the elbow and armpit (the brachial).
- Press gently with 2 fingers on inside of arm closest to you.
- Place thumb of same hand on outside of infant's upper arm.

**8**

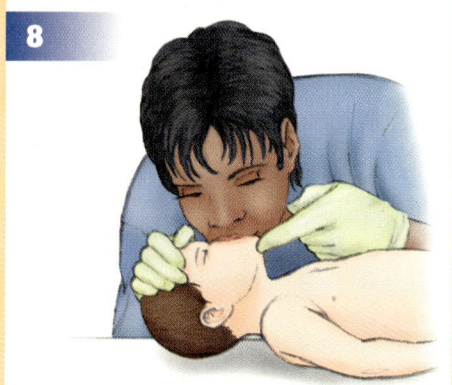

**Perform rescue procedures based on your pulse check.**

### If there is a pulse but no breathing

Give rescue breaths every 3 seconds. Use the same techniques for rescue breathing given in Step 6 but give only one breath. If you are alone, activate the EMS after the first minute. Every minute (20 breaths), stop and check the pulse to make sure there is one. Continue until:

- Infant starts breathing on his or her own.

OR

- Trained help, such as emergency medical technicians (EMTs), arrives and relieves you.

OR

- You are completely exhausted.

### If there is no pulse, give CPR

- Locate fingers' position.
  1. Maintain a head tilt.
  2. Imagine a line connecting the nipples.
  3. Place 3 fingers on sternum with index finger touching but below imaginary nipple line.
  4. Raise your index finger and use other 2 fingers for compression. If you feel the notch at the end of the sternum, move your fingers up a little.

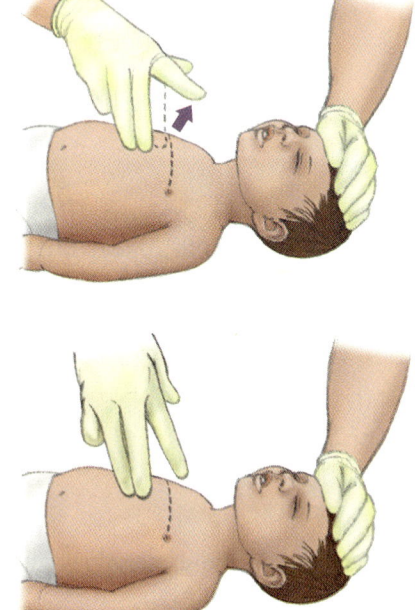

- Give 5 compressions.
  1. Do 5 chest compressions at rate of 100 per minute. Count as you push down, "one, two, three, four, five."
  2. Press sternum $\frac{1}{2}$ to 1 inch or about $\frac{1}{3}$ to $\frac{1}{2}$ of the depth of the chest.
  3. Keep fingers pointing across the infant's chest away from you. Keep fingers in contact with infant's chest.
  4. Maintain head tilt with hand nearest head on forehead.

**8**

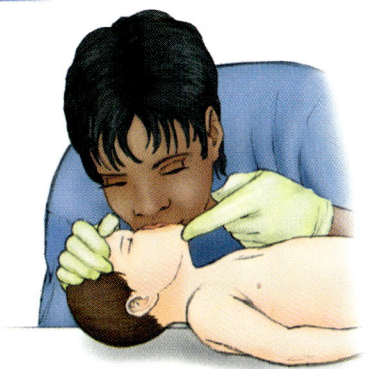

- Give 1 breath.
- Complete 20 cycles of 5 compressions and 1 breath (takes about 1 minute), then check the pulse. If you are alone, activate the EMS. If there is no pulse, restart CPR with chest compressions. Recheck the pulse every few minutes. If there is a pulse, give rescue breathing.
- Give CPR until:
  Infant revives.

OR

Trained help, such as emergency medical technicians (EMTs), arrives and relieves you.

OR

You are completely exhausted.

infant's lungs. As you remove your mouth, turn your head to the side to see if the infant's chest fell after each breath. For rescue breathing, breathe into the infant for the first second, count "one–one thousand" for the second, then take a breath yourself for the third second.

6. If a pulse is absent, begin chest compressions.
7. After one minute of CPR, activate the EMS if another rescuer has not.

# Airway Obstruction (Choking)

As discussed before, the airway may be partially or completely blocked. With a partial airway obstruction, an infant is able to make persistent coughing efforts that should not be hampered. If good air exchange becomes a poor exchange or poor air exchange occurs initially, the infant should be managed as having a complete airway obstruction. Poor air exchanges are indicated by ineffective coughing, high-pitched noises, breathing difficulty, and blueness of the lips and fingernail beds.

## Unconscious Infant

Choking management of a completely obstructed airway in an unconscious infant consists of the combination of back blows and chest thrusts. Abdominal thrusts are not advisable for infants because of possible injury to the abdominal organs. Finger sweeps of the mouth in an unconscious infant should be done only if the object can be seen. Finger sweeps should not be done with any conscious infant.

## Back Blows and Chest Thrusts

To perform back blows on an infant, straddle the infant facedown over your forearm. The infant's head should be lower than the trunk. Your hand should be around the jaw and neck of the infant giving support to the infant's head. For more support, rest your forearm under the infant on your thigh. Using the heel of the other hand, you are ready to give five rapid back blows between the infant's shoulder blades.

To give chest thrusts, turn the infant onto his or her back. Therefore, after delivering the five back blows, immediately place your free hand on the

back of the infant's head and neck while the other hand remains in place. Using both hands and forearms to sandwich the infant—one supporting the jaw, neck, and chest, and the other the back—turn the infant over. Once turned onto the back, the infant should be resting on your thigh. The infant's head should be lower than the trunk. With the infant positioned, give five chest thrusts in rapid succession. The thrusts are given to the sternum (between the nipples), using two fingers. The technique used to locate and perform chest thrusts is the same as that used to perform external chest compressions for CPR.

## Finger Sweeps

As stated earlier, do not perform blind finger sweeps of an infant. However, if the foreign body is visible, you should try to remove it, taking great care to avoid pushing it farther down into the airway.

The infant's mouth should be opened by means of the tongue-jaw lift. To perform the tongue-jaw lift, place your thumb in the infant's mouth over the tongue. Then grasp the infant's tongue and lower jaw between your thumb and fingers and lift them upward. If you can see a foreign body, sweep it out of the infant's mouth with your little finger.

## Unconscious Choking Victim Management

To help an unconscious choking infant, you should:

- Determine responsiveness.
- Call out for help.
- Open the infant's airway—use the head-tilt/chin-lift method.
- Determine if the infant is breathing by looking at the chest and listening for air coming out of the mouth and nose.
- Give two slow breaths. If the first breath does not go in, retilt the infant's head and try a second breath. *These breaths not going in indicates choking.*
- Give five back blows with the infant facing downward and head below the trunk.
- Give chest thrusts with the infant facing upward and head below the trunk.
- Using one hand, open the infant's mouth with the tongue-jaw lift. If a foreign object is seen, use the little finger of the other hand to finger sweep the mouth, and remove any reachable foreign body.

- Reposition the infant in a head-tilt/chin-lift position and give one breath.
- If unsuccessful, repeat the following steps until the airway is clear or until the infant becomes conscious: five back blows, five chest thrusts, look for object and if seen use a finger sweep, one breath.

## Conscious Infant

Help for a conscious infant also consists of the combined use of back blows and chest thrusts. These maneuvers are performed in the same manner as for an unconscious infant. They should be given when an infant has complete airway obstruction as evidenced by the inability to breathe, cough, or cry. No finger sweeps or rescue breaths should be attempted.

# Conscious Infant with Foreign Body Airway Obstruction (Choking)

**If infant is conscious and cannot cough, cry, or breathe . . .**

**1**

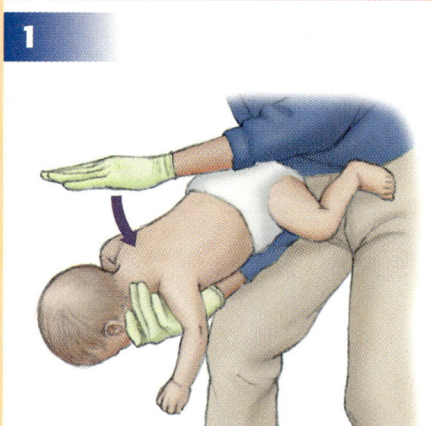

### Give up to 5 back blows

- Hold infant's head and neck with 1 hand by firmly supporting infant's jaw between your thumb and fingers.
- Lay infant face down over your forearm with head lower than his or her chest. Brace your forearm and infant against your thigh.
- Give up to 5 distinct and separate back blows between shoulder blades with the heel of your hand.

**2**

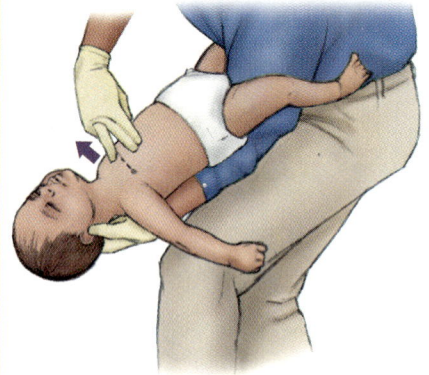

### Give up to 5 chest thrusts

- Support the back of infant's head.
- Sandwich infant between your hands and arms, turn on back, with head lower than chest. If you are small, you may need to support infant on your lap.
- Imagine a line connecting infant's nipples.
- Place 3 fingers on sternum with your ring finger next to imaginary nipple line on the infant's feet side.
- Lift your ring finger off chest. If you feel the notch at the end of the sternum, move your fingers up a little.
- Give up to 5 separate and distinct thrusts with index and middle fingers on sternum in a manner similar to CPR chest compressions, but at a slower rate.
- Keep fingers in contact with chest between chest thrusts.

**3**

### Repeat

- Give up to 5 back blows, then
- Give up to 5 chest thrusts until Infant becomes unconscious.

OR

   Object is expelled, and infant begins to breathe or cough forcefully.

**If infant is motionless . . .**

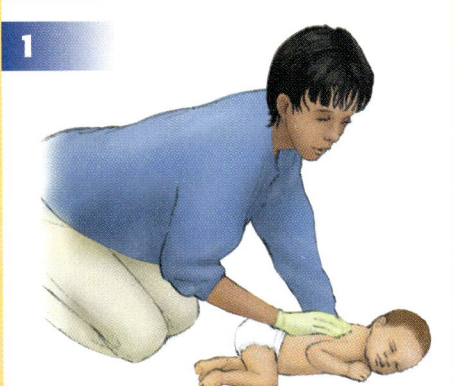

**1**

### Check responsiveness
- If spine injury is suspected, move infant only if absolutely necessary.
- Tap infant's shoulder.

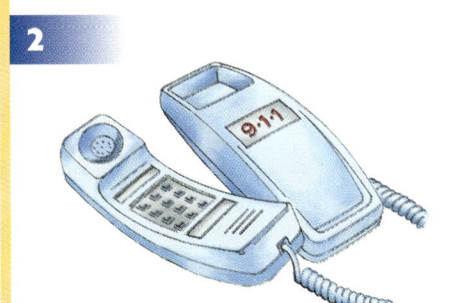

**2**

**Send bystander, if available, to activate EMS. If you are alone, resuscitate for 1 minute before activating EMS.**

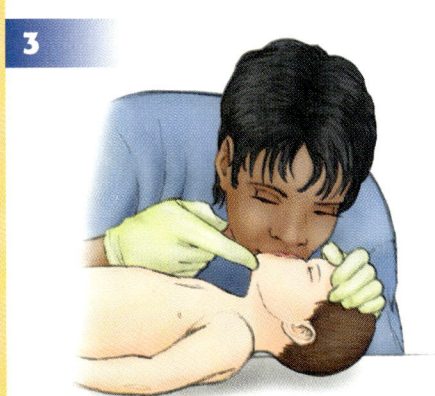

**3**

### Give 2 slow breaths
- Open the airway with head-tilt/chin-lift.
- Seal your mouth over infant's mouth and nose.
- Give 2 slow breaths (1 to 1½ seconds each).

If first breath did not go in, retilt the head and try 1 more slow breath.

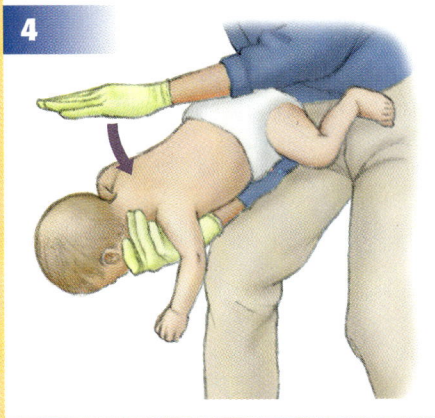

**4**

### Give up to 5 back blows
- Hold infant's head and neck with 1 hand by firmly supporting infant's jaw between your thumb and fingers.
- Lay infant face down over your forearm with head lower than chest. Brace your forearm and infant against your thigh.
- Give up to 5 distinct and separate back blows between shoulder blades with the heel of your hand.

**5**

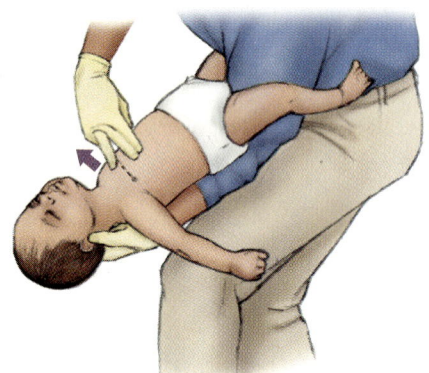

### Give up to 5 chest thrusts
- Support the back of infant's head.
- Sandwich infant between your hands and arms, then turn infant on back, with head lower than chest. If you are small, you may need to support infant on your lap.
- Imagine a line connecting infant's nipples.
- Place 3 fingers on sternum with your ring finger next to imaginary nipple line on the infant's feet side.
- Lift your ring finger off chest. If you feel the notch at the end of the sternum, move your fingers up a little.
- Give up to 5 separate and distinct thrusts with index and middle fingers on sternum in a manner similar to CPR chest compressions but at a slower rate.
- Keep fingers in contact with chest between chest thrusts.

**6**

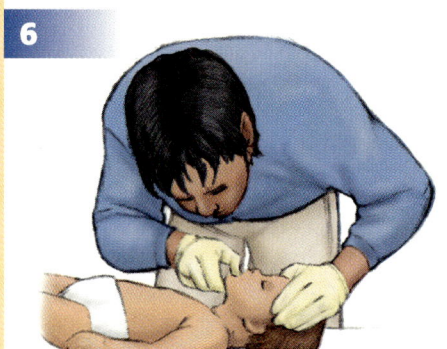

### Check mouth for foreign object
- Grasp both tongue and jaw between your thumb and fingers and lift up.
- If object is visible, remove it with a finger sweep by sliding your little finger of the other hand alongside cheek to base of tongue using a hooking action.
- Do *not* try to remove an object you cannot see (a "blind finger sweep").
- Do not push object deeper.

**7**

### Repeat
1. Give 1 slow breath.
2. Give up to 5 back blows.
3. Give up to 5 chest thrusts.
4. Check mouth for foreign object. If object is visible, use finger sweep.

Repeat until object is expelled or EMS arrives. If you are alone and after 1 minute the object has not been expelled, take infant with you and call the EMS.

# Infant Basic Life Support Proficiency Checklist

**S = self-check / P = partner check / I = instructor check**

## Infant Rescue Breathing

|  | S | P | I |
|---|---|---|---|
| 1. Check responsiveness. | ☐ | ☐ | ☐ |
| 2. Send a bystander, if available, to call EMS. | ☐ | ☐ | ☐ |
| 3. Roll infant onto back. | ☐ | ☐ | ☐ |
| 4. Airway open. | ☐ | ☐ | ☐ |
| 5. Breathing check. | ☐ | ☐ | ☐ |
| 6. 2 slow breaths. | ☐ | ☐ | ☐ |
| 7. Check pulse at brachial. | ☐ | ☐ | ☐ |
| 8. Rescue breathing (1 every 3 seconds). | ☐ | ☐ | ☐ |
| 9. If alone, call EMS after 1 minute. | ☐ | ☐ | ☐ |
| 10. Recheck pulse and breathing after first minute, then every few minutes. | ☐ | ☐ | ☐ |

## Infant CPR

|  | S | P | I |
|---|---|---|---|
| 1. Check responsiveness. | ☐ | ☐ | ☐ |
| 2. Send a bystander, if available, to call EMS. | ☐ | ☐ | ☐ |
| 3. Roll infant onto back. | ☐ | ☐ | ☐ |
| 4. Airway open. | ☐ | ☐ | ☐ |
| 5. Breathing check. | ☐ | ☐ | ☐ |
| 6. 2 slow breaths. | ☐ | ☐ | ☐ |
| 7. Check pulse at brachial. | ☐ | ☐ | ☐ |
| 8. Find fingers' position. | ☐ | ☐ | ☐ |
| 9. 5 chest compressions. | ☐ | ☐ | ☐ |
| 10. 1 slow breath. | ☐ | ☐ | ☐ |
| 11. Continue CPR for 1 minute (19 more cycles, for total of 20). | ☐ | ☐ | ☐ |
| 12. If alone, call EMS after 1 minute. | ☐ | ☐ | ☐ |
| 13. Recheck pulse. | ☐ | ☐ | ☐ |
| 14. Continue CPR (start with compressions). | ☐ | ☐ | ☐ |
| 15. Recheck pulse after first minute, then every few minutes. | ☐ | ☐ | ☐ |

## Conscious Infant Choking Management

|  | S | P | I |
|---|---|---|---|
| 1. Recognize choking. | ☐ | ☐ | ☐ |
| 2. Up to 5 back blows (head and face down). | ☐ | ☐ | ☐ |
| 3. Up to 5 chest thrusts (head down with face up). | ☐ | ☐ | ☐ |
| 4. Repeat Steps 2 and 3. | ☐ | ☐ | ☐ |

## Unconscious Infant Choking Management

|  | S | P | I |
|---|---|---|---|
| 1. Check responsiveness. | ☐ | ☐ | ☐ |
| 2. Send a bystander, if available, to call EMS. | ☐ | ☐ | ☐ |
| 3. Roll infant onto back. | ☐ | ☐ | ☐ |
| 4. Airway open. | ☐ | ☐ | ☐ |
| 5. Breathing check. | ☐ | ☐ | ☐ |
| 6. Try 2 slow breaths. (If first breath unsuccessful, retilt head and try 1 more breath.) | ☐ | ☐ | ☐ |
| 7. Up to 5 back blows (head and face down). | ☐ | ☐ | ☐ |
| 8. Up to 5 chest thrusts (head down and face up). | ☐ | ☐ | ☐ |
| 9. Check mouth for foreign object (finger sweep only if object is visible). | ☐ | ☐ | ☐ |
| 10. Try 1 slow breath. | ☐ | ☐ | ☐ |
| 11. Repeat sequence of 5 blows, 5 thrusts, mouth check, 1 breath. | ☐ | ☐ | ☐ |

# NOTES

# NOTES

# NOTES

# NOTES